COPING WITH BRAIN INJURY

MAGGIE RICH has enjoyed a career as, among other

# LINICLATE $\mathcal{B}$
## WESTERN ISLES LIBRARIES

Readers are requested to take great care of the item while in their possession, and to point out any defects that they may notice in them to the Librarian.
This item should be returned on or before the latest date stamped below, but an extention of the period of loan may be granted when desired.

| DATE OF RETURN | DATE OF RETURN | DATE OF RETURN |
|---|---|---|
| 20 NOV 2009 | | |

WITHDRAWN

# Overcoming Common Problems Series

*Selected titles*
A full list of titles is available from Sheldon Press,
36 Causton Street, London SW1P 4ST, and on our website at
www.sheldonpress.co.uk

# Overcoming Common Problems Series

**Coping with SAD**
Fiona Marshall and Peter Cheevers

**Coping with Snoring and Sleep Apnoea**
Jill Eckersley

**Coping with Stomach Ulcers**
Dr Tom Smith

**Coping with Strokes**
Dr Tom Smith

**Coping with Suicide**
Maggie Helen

**Coping with Teenagers**
Sarah Lawson

**Coping with Thyroid Problems**
Dr Joan Gomez

**Curing Arthritis – The Drug-Free Way**
Margaret Hills

**Curing Arthritis – More Ways to a Drug-Free Life**
Margaret Hills

**Curing Arthritis Diet Book**
Margaret Hills

**Curing Arthritis Exercise Book**
Margaret Hills and Janet Horwood

**Cystic Fibrosis – A Family Affair**
Jane Chumbley

**Depression at Work**
Vicky Maud

**Depressive Illness**
Dr Tim Cantopher

**Effortless Exercise**
Dr Caroline Shreeve

**Fertility**
Julie Reid

**The Fibromyalgia Healing Diet**
Christine Craggs-Hinton

**Getting a Good Night's Sleep**
Fiona Johnston

**The Good Stress Guide**
Mary Hartley

**Heal the Hurt: How to Forgive and Move On**
Dr Ann Macaskill

**Heart Attacks – Prevent and Survive**
Dr Tom Smith

**Helping Children Cope with Attention Deficit Disorder**
Dr Patricia Gilbert

**Helping Children Cope with Bullying**
Sarah Lawson

**Helping Children Cope with Change and Loss**
Rosemary Wells

**Helping Children Cope with Divorce**
Rosemary Wells

**Helping Children Cope with Grief**
Rosemary Wells

**Helping Children Cope with Stammering**
Jackie Turnbull and Trudy Stewart

**Helping Children Get the Most from School**
Sarah Lawson

**How to Accept Yourself**
Dr Windy Dryden

**How to Be Your Own Best Friend**
Dr Paul Hauck

**How to Cope with Anaemia**
Dr Joan Gomez

**How to Cope with Bulimia**
Dr Joan Gomez

**How to Cope with Stress**
Dr Peter Tyrer

**How to Enjoy Your Retirement**
Vicky Maud

**How to Improve Your Confidence**
Dr Kenneth Hambly

**How to Keep Your Cholesterol in Check**
Dr Robert Povey

**How to Lose Weight Without Dieting**
Mark Barker

**How to Make Yourself Miserable**
Dr Windy Dryden

**How to Pass Your Driving Test**
Donald Ridland

**How to Stand up for Yourself**
Dr Paul Hauck

**How to Stick to a Diet**
Deborah Steinberg and Dr Windy Dryden

**How to Stop Worrying**
Dr Frank Tallis

**The How to Study Book**
Alan Brown

**How to Succeed as a Single Parent**
Carole Baldock

**How to Untangle Your Emotional Knots**
Dr Windy Dryden and Jack Gordon

**Hysterectomy**
Suzie Hayman

# Overcoming Common Problems Series

**Overcoming Common Problems**

# Coping with Brain Injury

How to Help after Accidents, Stroke and Illness

## Maggie Rich

**sheldon** PRESS

First published in Great Britain in 2005

Sheldon Press
36 Causton Street
London SW1P 4ST

*British Library Cataloguing-in-Publication Data*

A catalogue record for this book is available from the British Library

ISBN 0–85969–924–2

1 3 5 7 9 10 8 6 4 2

Typeset by Deltatype Limited, Birkenhead, Merseyside
Printed in Great Britain by Ashford Colour Press

For others who find themselves living closely alongside a brain injury, this book is intended as an encouraging – if inadequate – hug.

# Contents

# Introduction: Crash landing

So someone close to you has had a brain injury. Doubtless the first few days – perhaps a good many more – have passed in a blur of confusion as you have tried to absorb the shock and take in what has happened. You will have been engaged in a whirl of activity, involving hospitals, doctors, phone calls, family and friends, as well as coping with practical arrangements for the adjustment of your daily routine – looking after the needs of children, negotiating absence from work, remembering to feed the dog and all the rest of it.

By the time you pick up this book, those earliest days will probably be behind you. The brain injury has happened. Whether this injury has been 'traumatic' (the result of a physical blow to the head, suffered in a fall or a car crash, for example) or the result of a stroke, a brain haemorrhage or an infection such as encephalitis, the extent of the physical damage to the brain will have been assessed. But the nature and extent of the difficulties that will arise from that injury will take a lot longer to become clear.

Although research in this area is now moving on quickly, the workings of the brain are still poorly understood. Sometimes it is possible to predict particular difficulties that will or will not arise when the injury is confined to one part of the brain. We know, for example, that a stroke on the right side of the brain is likely to affect speech, while a stroke on the left side will not. Experts are aware of the rough location of various other functions in the brain. But because the network of connections within the brain is so very complex, if the damage to the brain is spread over a wide area, or is patchy in several areas, it is not at all easy to predict accurately or helpfully the future outcome.

Added to that, there have been cases where a part of the brain with a specific purpose was damaged and over time new pathways have developed in the brain so as to bypass the damage and recover the function. Again, this ability of the brain to renew itself is poorly understood and should certainly not be relied upon.

As far as the recovery of your loved one is concerned, two things seem certain. The doctors and specialists advising you are likely to err on the side of caution in any predictions they might make. And the brain is very slow to heal.

It may yet be a long while before you know what sort of recovery your loved one might make. They may eventually make a full recovery and be totally independent. They may regain their physical abilities but have ongoing problems with one or more of a whole range of brain functions: speech, for example, or memory, or controlling their emotions. They may regain the appearance of someone perfectly able, but in fact be very handicapped and unable to function without support. Or they may only make slight progress and regain very little in the way of either physical or mental ability.

'Two years' is often quoted as the length of time it takes for the brain to heal after injury. Learn to treat this with caution. Two years may be roughly the length of time necessary for brain tissue to heal physically. But, always depending on the particular extent and areas of damage and assuming that significant recovery has already been made, the brain's ability to adjust to a damaged part and to develop ways of compensating for that damage can mean that progress continues beyond that time.

Imagine, for example, that you have injured your wrist. In the first place there might be swelling and bruising, but this will reduce and disappear quite quickly. After a certain length of time, say three months, you may realize that your wrist is not actually going to get any better. During those three months you have been unable to turn on a tap or hold a heavy kettle with that hand. You've had to fill the kettle by setting it down in the sink so as to turn the tap on with your good hand. But once you admit that your damaged wrist is not going to get any better, you may well discover that you can develop a new way of turning on the tap by pulling from your elbow instead of your wrist. In a similar way, the brain may itself discover ways to adapt so as to work round its damaged parts and make the best of things.

But alongside and within all these considerations, it's important to remember that your loved one is not the only one who has suffered this brain injury. It will take time for you too to recover: to get over the shock of it all, to mourn the loss that you have suffered, to adjust to the new circumstances of your life, and to learn to relate to a new friend or family member.

We none of us exist in a vacuum. Shock waves will go out from this brain injury – the immediate victim, their partner, members of their family, friends, work colleagues – all will have a greater or lesser degree of adjustment to make. And once this has happened to you, it may well surprise you how often you come across others in a similar situation. You may wonder where they have all suddenly appeared from. Well, they were there before – it's just the connection with you that is new and makes their presence register.

Around 11,000 people in the UK every year suffer a severe head injury, rendering them unconscious for six hours or longer. After five years only 15 per cent of these people will have been able to return to their former occupation.

Advances in medical science raced ahead in the last third of the twentieth century. Before that, many who now survive brain injuries would undoubtedly have died. More and more people are living with brain injury, Unfortunately it has taken our society some considerable time to catch up with this fact. Services for the brain injured are improving but are still a bit patchy around the UK.

And so this book has several purposes. To some extent it can be used as a starting point for practical advice, information and ideas, as a reference for opportunities in rehabilitation and therapies and perhaps as an informal yardstick for good practice in some areas.

But perhaps its primary aim is to serve as a source of some emotional support for your journey. Friends, family, even professional and semi-professional sources of support and a listening ear can be of great benefit. But over an extended period of time it can be difficult to go back to the same person again and again, and perhaps even harder to have to start from the beginning with someone new. At times like these, I hope this book might be able to say to you, 'You are not alone. There are many out there who understand. Many who are engaged in the same struggle. The struggle is worthwhile. Rest awhile, gather up your resources, and start again.'

# 1

## The different types of brain injury

Just like any other cells in the body, brain cells need oxygen in order to live – the oxygen that is carried around the body in the blood supply. If the supply of blood to the brain – or part of the brain – is lowered or blocked by whatever cause, brain cells are going to be damaged, and will eventually die if the blockage continues.

There is a range of incidents that can reduce or block the blood supply in the brain, and these are generally divided into two groups: traumatic brain injury, and other types of brain injury.

A *traumatic brain injury (TBI)* is an injury that results from a blow to the head. There may be a visible wound to the head, with obvious damage to blood vessels, so that blood is seen to be seeping or pouring out. But the injury does not have to be visible. Because the brain is encased in a solid skull, any blow to the head can cause the brain to move suddenly and injure itself against the inside of the hard skull. (Think of an egg inside a tin being whacked by a mallet.) Bleeding and swelling will then occur inside the skull, so that even without an apparent wound to the head, the blood supply to parts of the brain will have been affected beyond the damaged blood vessels. In fact, the worst of the injury is often caused not by the actual wound but by the swelling that comes afterwards; swollen brain tissue has nowhere to go to, but can only press against the hard skull causing further damage to itself.

Injury to the brain as the result of a TBI may be fairly localized. But it is often the case that there are two specific areas of damage. The first, and the more serious, will be beneath the point where the blow has directly impacted on the head. The second area of damage will be on the opposite side of the brain, where the brain's sudden movement in response to the impact has caused it to knock against the hard casing of the skull.

A TBI may result from something as simple as a bang on the head on getting into a car or going through a low doorway, to something less common such as a fall from a height, an attack with a heavy instrument in a mugging, or a head wound in a serious car crash. TBIs often used to be called 'head injuries' but people are moving

1

away from that term now because, whether or not there is a visible wound to the head, it is the injury to the brain inside the head that has the serious consequences.

## Other types of acquired brain injury

A *stroke* (otherwise known as a cerebrovascular accident or CVA) is the commonest cause of brain injury, and occurs when a blood vessel becomes blocked by a blood clot, or becomes so narrowed that blood cannot get through. In both situations, brain cells will die beyond the obstruction because of lack of oxygen.

A *brain haemorrhage* is bleeding inside the brain from a burst blood vessel. The blood leaks out into the brain tissue or into the cavity between the brain and the skull. In this case, injury is caused not only by the loss of blood supply to cells, but by a build-up of pressure on cells as blood (continuing to be pumped up from the heart) collects in what is a very restricted space within the skull.

*Encephalitis* means, simply, an inflammation of the brain and is the result of an infection, usually a virus. This tracks up from the nose and mouth and into the brain along nerve fibres, which split and divide to reach across into all the different areas, where it attacks the cells. Because of this, brain damage caused by encephalitis may be more scattered than that resulting from the other types of injury.

*Anoxia* is an interruption in the supply of oxygen to the brain from any other cause, such as cardiac arrest, an anaesthetic accident, near drowning or carbon monoxide poisoning.

## Mild, moderate and severe brain injury

Two particular symptoms are used to define the severity of a brain injury: loss of consciousness and post-traumatic amnesia (PTA). Post-traumatic amnesia is the period of time after an injury during which a person is confused and disorientated. The longer these two symptoms last, the more severe the brain injury is considered to be.

So a *mild* brain injury is one in which there is no loss of consciousness at all, or the person is knocked out for just a few minutes, and remains dizzy or dazed and perhaps feeling sick for a little while longer. In a *moderate* brain injury, loss of consciousness lasts for between 15 minutes and 6 hours and post-traumatic amnesia lasts for up to 24 hours after that. If loss of consciousness lasts for more than 6 hours and post-traumatic amnesia for more than 24 hours, the brain injury is considered *severe*.

These terms may help us in predicting the length of time that the physical recovery of the brain might take. However, they don't necessarily tell us very much about the level of difficulty that people may be left with in their day-to-day lives as a result of the injury.

# 2

# What to expect of the patient

## *Lowered consciousness and coma*

Where the brain injury has been traumatic, especially if we can see a wound and loss of blood, we naturally expect a 'lowered consciousness'. Even if the person is not knocked unconscious, they may suffer from dizziness or nausea, become drowsy with slow or slurred speech, have a lack of awareness of what is going on around them and difficulty in recollecting what has happened to them recently.

When the injury is from another cause it is quite likely that, along with a headache perhaps, these sorts of symptoms are the first indication to those around that something is not as it should be. Written down starkly on the page they look very obvious, but if they appear gradually over a number of days they might be less noticeable than you think. And it may simply be the case that the person drifts into sleeping more, and more heavily than usual.

If you consider what the brain is struggling to cope with – attack in the form of trauma or infection, loss of blood, lack of oxygen – an alteration in the level of consciousness is not at all surprising. Something has to give in order to allow the brain to focus on maintaining the essential functions of the heart and lungs.

Coma may come about suddenly – or gradually over a period of days. It is considered to be the lowest level of consciousness, a state of unresponsiveness from which someone cannot at present be aroused. In fact it is not in itself one level of consciousness but a range of levels that merge into one another. The depth of a coma is measured according to the Glasgow Coma Scale, a rating of 3 to 15 being given to describe how much of a response is made when the patient is asked to open their eyes, to move a part of the body (a motor response) and to speak (a verbal response). The lower the number the deeper is the coma.

This is a frightening time for family and friends. Coma is a peculiar state, relished by soap operas and sentimental films for its dramatic power. You will naturally be anxious about the patient, and desperate for them to communicate to you something of how they are.

Sometimes drugs are used to stop the patient moving about so as to reduce irritation to the brain, and these can have the effect of making the coma seem deeper than it actually is. It's also likely that such patients will be wired up to various monitors to provide continuous information about their condition. All of this adds to the abnormality of the situation and the anxiety of those visiting.

It is understandable for you to want to hurry the patient through this period as quickly as possible. But it might be as well, if you can, to try to see the coma as part of the natural process, allowing the brain to conserve energy for the essentials. Perhaps for a while it needs to focus on the fighting of infection, the recovery from trauma, to begin to adjust to the injury and to embark on the healing process – rather than on giving you the reassurance that you so desperately want. Try to be patient.

Some hospitals encourage the use of 'coma arousal programmes'. These include planned periods in which the patient is stimulated by touch, sound, taste or smell, alternated with periods of complete rest. It is now well known that, although coma patients seem to be completely unaware of what is happening around them, this can be far from the case. So do at least talk to your loved one, letting them know that you care, that they are being well looked after, telling them of any progress they have made, encouraging them. But don't expect their emergence from the coma to be as it is in the films, a sudden opening of the eyes, a 'Where am I?' and all is immediately – or very soon – well. Coming out of coma is a gradual process and will take a period of several days at least, if not longer.

One particular fear related to coma is that the person may in fact not emerge. 'Persistent vegetative state' or PVS is an ongoing state of reduced consciousness, in which the person remains alive, maintaining the essential functions of heart and lungs without mechanical help, but trapped in this state of unresponsiveness. It is a rare condition; at any one time in the UK there are usually fewer than 100 people living in this state.

## Confusion and behavioural changes

Along with a slightly lowered consciousness, confusion and behavioural changes are to be expected. After all, if someone has less awareness or understanding of what is going on around them, or is having difficulty recalling what they have been doing, they are likely to seem muddled. Try to put yourself in their shoes for a moment. Imagine the feeling of not understanding properly what is going on around you and the sensation of not being able to engage properly with other people. It's the stuff of nightmares. No wonder if a normally placid and unshakeable person becomes rattled and short-tempered, if only out of natural alarm and anxiety as to what might be happening to them.

But the behavioural changes may relate not just to the way the person is responding to what is happening to them, but to changes taking place within the brain itself. For example, a person may suddenly begin to walk in an unusual way for no apparent reason, or develop a twitch. Or they may do things that they wouldn't normally do, that seem very strange to members of their family, such as being adamant they won't go out without a hat when they haven't worn one for years, or drinking five cups of coffee one morning when last week they'd decided to give it up as bad for them. Of course, human behaviour is often 'odd' in this way and doesn't necessarily mean a brain injury!

Confusion too covers a whole spectrum, from being slightly muddle-headed, to being unable to distinguish between hot water and cold, to spreading Marmite on a sheet of newspaper instead of a slice of bread. The person who is *very* confused is visibly so, and I don't mean the picture of confusion where someone's face is screwed up in puzzlement with a finger to their lips as they try to think. The very confused person appears completely separate from their environment, apparently only able to engage with it as if through a thick fog.

*Confabulation* is the term used for the way in which patients with memory disorders can produce false memories. In answering a question from you they may go off on a complete flight of fantasy, involving memories that simply cannot be correct. They may rove over a number of themes, producing very bizarre stories, which nevertheless have the ring of plausibility. The patient is unaware that they are producing false memories and, although they may start from a point of fact, it is often difficult for the listener to identify where fact and fantasy meet. Confabulation can be disorientating for all concerned and distressing for relatives and carers, but it often settles with time.

## Seizures or fits

Seizures take a range of forms, some more alarming than others. Most seizures last somewhere between a few seconds and a few minutes, and stop naturally. The mildest type of seizure, the *absence*, takes the form of the person simply 'going blank' for a few moments, during which they will be still and fail to respond to others.

*Partial seizures* are so-called because they involve only a part of the brain, and in this type of seizure the person may experience sudden feelings of joy or sadness, or sudden sensations of smell, hearing or vision. In a *complex partial seizure*, the person may behave in a strange, repetitive way; for example they may blink repeatedly, or keep moving an arm or a leg in a particular way, without being able to stop themselves.

The *generalized seizure*, a seizure that spreads to involve the whole of the brain, is probably more familiar to us. In this type of seizure the person may lose consciousness, fall, have jerking muscles all over the body, or stare into space and lose contact with reality for a short time. This is the type of seizure that we associate with epilepsy; and epilepsy in fact means simply the ongoing experience of seizures.

A seizure occurs when there is unusual electrical activity going on in the brain. The nerve cells that carry impulses around the brain develop into complex webs of 'wires'. When they are damaged and these pathways are broken, the brain works to repair itself. But it may make new abnormal connections – it may 'wire itself up wrongly' – and it is these that can cause seizures or fits.

It is common for someone who has suffered a brain injury to develop seizures, and epilepsy can be a permanent result of brain injury (particularly in children). But often, as the brain sorts itself out after injury and begins to heal, the abnormal electrical activity begins to settle down, seizures become less frequent, and will hopefully become a thing of the past.

In the meantime, there are many drugs that are used to control epilepsy. It may, however, take a considerable period of trial and error in order to discover the one that is most effective for this particular individual, and the least troublesome in its side effects.

# 3

# What to expect in terms of treatment

## Intensive care

Depending of course on the severity of the injury, intensive care may be necessary. The brain controls all the bodily functions: breathing, the movement of muscles both voluntary (such as in the hand) and involuntary (such as in the lungs), the heart rate, the sending of chemical messages (hormones) around the body, the control of the body's temperature, and so on. In the case of a serious injury, it may well be necessary for some of these functions to be controlled artificially in order to keep the person alive. Or the medical team may consider it advisable to keep the person under very close observation in case their condition deteriorates and artificial intervention becomes necessary.

Only in the intensive care ward, where each patient has their own one-to-one nurse, can such close observation be maintained from minute to minute around the clock. Resources are available on this ward for every patient to have heart rate, breathing and body temperature closely monitored, so that action can be immediate if anything takes a turn for the worse. Drugs can be given via a 'line' or tube that is constantly in place. Everything is set up for the best of care.

The role of friends and family in the patient's recovery is fully appreciated nowadays. You will be positively welcomed at the bedside although there may be a strict hygiene procedure to go through first. Be ready to move out of the way quickly if necessary, and don't be impatient if you are asked to move to the waiting room for a period while treatment is carried out. Such requests are always made either for the sake of giving the best nursing care, or to save you unnecessary distress.

## Investigative procedures

### Brain scans

In the early days and perhaps also at various stages during recovery one or more means of looking at the brain to assess the physical

9

damage is likely to be used. There are several types of *brain scan* around nowadays and which one is used will depend partly on the equipment that the particular hospital has available, and partly on the reason for which a scan is felt to be desirable. The *computerized tomography (CT) scan* (also known as a CAT (computerized axial tomography) scan) uses X-rays to take a picture of the brain in 'slices' at different levels, giving a very detailed picture of the brain's condition and a much clearer image than an ordinary X-ray could possibly provide. The patient lies on a table which an operator moves forward and back through the ring-shaped scanner in order to get an image of the required part of the body. It is a painless procedure, apart from the fact that the patient has to lie still on a hard surface for perhaps half an hour. A sedative might be given to make this easier.

The *magnetic resonance imaging (MRI) scan* is performed by a similar machine to the CAT scan, but the ring is longer – more of a tube. In whole body scans, the patient moves all the way through the tube, but when just the brain is being scanned only the head needs to be within the tube. The scanner uses a very powerful magnet to build up detailed images of the brain, again in slices. The radiographer sits behind a screen and can see and hear the patient at all times. Different types of tissue show up in different colours on the screen, so a very detailed image can be acquired. There are no known side effects to this procedure.

Other types of scan less commonly used include the *positron emission tomography (PET) scan* and the *single photon emission computerized tomography (SPECT) scan*. The PET scan is only rarely available and in connection with brain injury is helpful only in the assessment of epilepsy. In the SPECT scan a radioactive chemical is given to the patient in an intravenous injection, and this allows the blood supply in the brain to be mapped, showing areas of damage.

One other, rather different way of looking at what's going on in the brain is the *electroencephalogram (EEG)*. This machine doesn't give a picture of the brain as such, but is used to measure electrical activity within the brain. Electrodes are attached to the scalp and a visual representation of the brain's activity will appear on the monitor to which they are wired up.

A *lumbar puncture*, a means of taking a sample of the fluid which surrounds the brain and the spinal column, may well be performed if the cause of the brain malfunction is not obvious. It can diagnose or rule out meningitis. A hollow needle is inserted between two of the vertebrae in the spine and a small amount of fluid drawn out under local anaesthetic. The presence of blood in the fluid will signify a haemorrhage, while an increased level of white blood cells will indicate the presence of an infection. The hospital laboratory will analyse the specimen thoroughly and try to grow a culture from it in order to discover the particular organism behind the infection.

## Keeping the body in balance

Thanks to hospital dramas on television we are fairly well accustomed to the sight of many of the more standard hospital procedures, such as the setting up of a *drip*, properly known as an intravenous infusion. The drip is a means of getting fluid and calories into the body and of maintaining the balance of the body salts, and can also be used as a route for drug treatments.

The normal way for the brain to express the body's need for fluid is via the sensation of thirst. While thirst cannot be expressed, or while fluid cannot be taken by mouth, the patient's fluid intake and output (via urine, diarrhoea – a side effect of many drugs – and any ongoing bleeding) must be carefully measured on a daily basis to prevent dehydration.

The *catheter*, as well as being a means of preventing the discomfort of wet sheets and the bedsores that would result, is also a useful tool in this process. It is simply a tube that is passed up the urethra and into the bladder, to allow the urine to drain freely into a bag, calibrated for measurement. The catheter must be inserted into the body under sterile conditions so as to prevent any infection being introduced at the same time. Once in, the inflation of a small balloon should keep the catheter in place. However, it is not unknown for it to become dislodged or even be yanked out by a confused patient.

## Treatment with drugs

Depending on the type of brain injury and the stage in the treatment process, a whole array of medications may be given, or none. Antibiotics and antivirals for the control of infection, anticoagulants to prevent clots, drugs to reduce the swelling in the brain, to minimize seizures, to counteract the side effects of other drugs, and so on.

Among those of us who are outside the medical profession, one of two reactions to such treatment is likely – or else a mixture of both. You may be horrified at the thought of so many chemicals being pumped into your loved one's body. Or you may put all your faith in medical drugs, and feel confident that something somewhere will bring about the desired result.

Probably the most helpful attitude lies somewhere between these two. Drugs are best regarded as something like a 'necessary evil'. Most people would prefer to do without drugs, but at times like this they cannot safely be avoided. Medical staff may seem rather casual about their use, but this is simply because they are part and parcel of their daily experience, not because they resort to them without due care and consideration, especially of their side effects. Don't expect that treatment of a serious brain injury (from whatever cause) is likely to proceed without the use of drugs. But don't suppose either that there is a drug to solve every problem.

You don't nowadays have to trust blindly in the doctors caring for the injured person. You are free to ask for as much information as you want and to discuss the various treatment options, being sensitive though to the call of other patients on the doctor's time. The Internet can be a great source of information if you really want to understand what is going on and if you don't have access at home you can always use the public library. But do be aware that this sort of exploration can sap your energy, almost without you noticing; you may feel it is worth trusting the experts and conserving that energy for other vital tasks.

## Operative procedures

The vast majority of people who suffer a serious traumatic brain injury will need no surgical treatment (to the head) other than the stitching up of the wound. Operations on the brain are generally performed for the removal of a clot or a tumour, for the draining of a collection of blood or fluid that is causing excessive pressure, or for the removal of an aneurysm or problematic blood vessel. For whatever reason surgery is being considered, it will be only in a situation of necessity, and the surgeon will always be prepared (assuming the operation is not immediately urgent) to explain it to you and to offer reassurance can. If you need it explaining more than once, don't be embarrassed to ask; for most people, the first thought of surgery on the brain is so upsetting that little if any of the more detailed information given after this is likely to be taken in.

A procedure that is quite likely in a severe brain injury is the performance of a *tracheostomy*. When the patient first became unconscious a simple airway tube may have been used, like those used after any operation under general anaesthetic, that goes through the mouth and down over the back of the tongue, to prevent the tongue falling back over the throat and choking the patient. A tracheostomy is a safer and more comfortable arrangement over a longer period of time for making sure that the airway remains open. A hole is made through the front of the neck and into the trachea or windpipe, and a tube inserted to keep this open.

This tube can then be attached to the ventilator or ventilating machine which can manage the patient's breathing when necessary. The brain controls breathing, just like every other bodily function. When the brain has been injured there is a very real risk that it might 'forget' to breathe, so for a time it makes sense to relieve it of that job.

As the patient begins to recover, the ventilator can be disconnected for periods, during which the patient will breathe through the tube in their neck. As the individual recovers further, a cap can be put onto this tube for gradually increasing periods of time so the patient can regain control and strength of the muscles in the neck that assist breathing. While there is an open tube in the trachea, the patient cannot use their voice, but capping of the tube allows them to speak again.

One other operation that may need to be performed, much later, is a *gastrostomy*, the making of a hole directly into the stomach for the purpose of feeding. The unconscious patient will be 'fed' by means of an intravenous infusion, giving the necessary calories in the simplest way for the body to cope with them. Later, if the patient cannot manage eating safely, they may be fed liquidized food via a nasogastric tube, which ensures that, even if the patient does not have a secure cough reflex or the ability to swallow, the food goes

13

down into the stomach. If we can't swallow we may inhale food into our windpipe, and if the cough reflex is not present, food will end up in the lungs where it will set up an infection. When a very confused patient is forever pulling out a nasogastric tube, the gastrostomy may provide the best solution, though as a last resort.

# 4

# The role of the professionals

## *Nurses*

A bewildering array of professionals stalks the ward nowadays, particularly in the case of something as complicated as a brain injury. Nevertheless, the *nursing team* is likely to be your most immediate point of contact, and their expertise in carrying out routine procedures in the hour-to-hour and day-to-day care of the patient will be invaluable. In the intensive care ward, each patient has their own nurse treating them on a one-to-one basis. In other wards it is usual practice for each patient to have their own *named nurse*. This nurse has a particular responsibility to be properly familiar with the patient's condition and its treatment, to get to know them – and the family – as individuals and to liaise between the various members of staff. It is likely to be this person, or their superior, the *ward sister*, who will be able to answer your questions or calm your worries.

The nurses are responsible for looking after the whole person, and they are experts in the sort of treatment involved with the complete range of the many and varied conditions that land people in hospital. For example, they understand the need to take regular observations of pulse, temperature and blood pressure and what the various changes in these might mean. They are aware of the needs of the patient to be kept clean and dry, and to be turned regularly if they are unable to turn themselves, to prevent the breakdown of the skin into bedsores. They are skilled at giving injections, setting up drips, inserting catheters, administering suppositories . . . and many other treatments and procedures. The junior nurses are likely to be students, working through a series of placements in a variety of wards in order to gain some experience of a range of conditions. The more senior nursing staff will probably have been on the ward longer and may well have several years' experience of nursing patients with brain injury or related conditions.

## *Doctors*

While the senior nurses in particular should have a clear and full understanding of the treatment and be able to answer most if not all of your questions, it is the *consultant*, or the *registrar* under them, who actually decides what treatment should be given. The consultant is the most senior doctor, the registrar their assistant, and the next step down in the hierarchy is the houseman, who is training under them. The consultant you are dealing with may belong to a range of disciplines. They may be a *consultant in medicine* (a specialist in conditions that are treated with drugs), a *consultant neurologist* (a specialist in conditions that affect the nervous system), a *surgeon* (a specialist in surgical operations) or a *neurosurgeon* (a specialist in operations on the brain or spinal cord). The type of consultant involved in your case will depend largely on the type of brain injury that your loved one has suffered and how it is to be treated. But it will also depend to some extent on the way the staffing of this particular hospital or healthcare trust is structured, as well as on the availability of particular specialists within the National Health Service at any one time. Neurologists and neurosurgeons are fairly rare breeds, for example, and it may be that the patient will need to be moved to another hospital in order to receive expert oversight more easily.

Complaints about healthcare in the UK are very common, but when the chips are really down we begin to appreciate how fortunate we are. That said, don't just accept things blindly; it is important that you understand what is going on, why certain decisions are being made, and that they are being made with your loved one's best interests at heart. There may be some difficult issues to balance; it's not always that ethical, practical and medical considerations fall neatly into line, although they do tend to fall into a fairly clear order of priority when the odds are stacking up. You should feel able to discuss *all* your concerns with the hospital staff. You are the one who knows the patient as an individual, a fully blown personality, who may have had opinions to express about the situation they find themselves in now. The hospital staff are there to treat the whole person; not only is your relationship with the patient clearly a part of the picture, but you are also likely to have valuable information to contribute.

# *Therapists*

Apart from the medical and/or surgical team, the therapists are important early players in the field of brain injury. The *physiotherapist* is likely to have been visiting almost from the point of admission, passively exercising limbs to prevent them wasting through lack of use. You are likely to be recruited to help with this task, as it is a case of the more the better, and it is good that you can feel of practical help as you maintain your vigil – if you do. The physio is also responsible for keeping the lungs clear while the patient is lying down so much; any build-up of mucus in the chest could put the patient at risk of infection. As time passes and assuming the patient regains consciousness and mental capacity, the physio will be involved in helping them overcome paralysis to regain full control of their limbs, to learn to walk again, to maintain a good posture, and to develop full physical potential through exercise and simple sporting activity.

Another important therapist, who will work closely alongside the physio in some settings, is the *occupational therapist*. It's commonly thought that occupational therapy is about giving the patient things to do – keeping them usefully occupied. But, much more importantly, it is actually concerned with helping them regain the ability to do the things that are necessary for day-to-day life. The occupational therapist can't work with the patient until they have returned to consciousness and have some awareness (however confused) of themselves. She will assess their ability to carry out a whole range of 'activities of daily living' – things like going up and down stairs, getting dressed, making a cup of tea, getting in and out of bed – and she will give a score to the level of their ability. Over many weeks she will then work on these activities, breaking them down into the minutest segments necessary for their smooth running. So, for example, if going up stairs is a problem, it may be to do with an inability to flex the foot. If feeding themselves is a problem, it may actually be to do with the type of chair being used – better posture from a tilted stool might improve the situation over a period of some weeks. Through a combination of training, repetition and the use of specialized equipment, the therapist will work to improve the patient's independence and increase the score in these tasks. It will be a slow process, but it can bring extraordinary results. The

17

occupational therapist also has expert knowledge of a whole range of adaptive and remedial equipment, from wheelchairs and seats, through splints designed to open up clawed hands, to specialized cutlery and kitchen aids.

The *speech and language therapist* is another important member of the therapy team, although her first involvement with the patient will strictly speaking have nothing to do with either speech or language. She is first responsible for assessing the patient's ability to swallow, along with the purely physical state of the mouth and upper throat. Her first job, soon after the patient has emerged from coma, or soon after the stroke, will be to work on desensitizing the mouth. The sensitivity of the mouth is often increased at this time, and the therapist will work to reduce this; a simple process of touching and stroking different areas of the mouth and tongue with cotton buds. Related to this, the speech therapist is also responsible for assessing the patient's ability to swallow. Only once this instinctive reaction has been regained is it safe for the patient to take food or drink by mouth again.

Later, the speech and language therapist will spend time with the patient working on their ability to communicate. The use of this therapist's full title is significant. Speech therapy, like physiotherapy and occupational therapy, is a way of working on the body so as to have an educational impact on the brain. In other words, by repetitive training the brain learns how to carry out an action, whether that is walking, moving a spoon to the mouth, or in this case shaping the mouth in order to produce the necessary sounds for speech. Language therapy work has a more direct involvement with the brain itself, working with the deeper concepts of language as it is formulated in the mind.

There is a whole range of communication skills that can be damaged by a brain injury. Some of these are verbal (to do with words) and some non-verbal. Some will be to do with expression (the communication of thoughts and feelings) and some to do with comprehension (the understanding of what is being said). It's not easy for the layperson to separate the two, since we mostly communicate our understanding through our speech. But the speech and language therapist's training enables her, using comprehensive assessments, to separate out the different strands of language and ascertain what the specific difficulties are. She will then prescribe particular exercises to help overcome these with practice. At this point, you may well be able to help by offering the extra practice between sessions that can maximize progress.

For the *cognitive therapist* to be of help the patient will need to have regained some awareness of their own patterns of behaviour, or at least the ability to recognize these when they are drawn to their attention. That's because cognitive therapy is about working with your own modes of thought in order to change the way you behave. Perhaps the most common example would be in anger management. People who have suffered a brain injury often have difficulty in controlling a range of emotions. Of these, anger is the one that can get people into serious trouble and probably is also the most harmful to relationships, and so perhaps has the most detrimental effect on someone's life. In training someone to manage their anger, the cognitive therapist would help them first to identify the various things that trigger an outburst, and the normal progress of feelings and behaviours that contribute to the overall pattern of the angry reaction. They will then suggest ways that an individual may react differently, or block an outburst – by such simple means, perhaps, as counting from one to ten before shouting in anger. Through a process of acting out situations, practising and reviewing how the individual is managing to bring changes into effect, real differences can be made over a period of time. The cognitive therapist is becoming a more common team member in a rehabilitation setting, but is also someone it may be appropriate to seek help from further down the line (via the GP), if problematic behaviours get in the way of a settled home life for – or with – a brain injured individual.

Becoming more common now in certain settings is the use of *rehabilitation assistants*. These members of staff have been trained in the carrying-out of a range of therapeutic procedures, but have not done all the study necessary to lead to a professional qualification and don't necessarily understand fully the theory behind the practice. They will work under the supervision of a fully qualified therapist in one or more disciplines. The professionally qualified therapist will decide what exercises (mental or physical) will help the patient's condition, will ensure that the assistant is trained in carrying these out properly and will keep an interested eye on the patient's progress without being present at every session. Assistants are of course more economical to employ, but provided the system is running properly, there should be no loss of expertise in the patient's therapeutic care.

## Other specialists

Your loved one may well be referred to other specialist professionals during the course of their care and rehabilitation. The *neuropsychologist* is trained to identify the particular difficulties of thinking that have resulted from brain damage. They focus on areas such as vision, attention, memory, language and the so-called 'executive functions' of the brain. Executive functions are things like planning, moving flexibly from one task to another and back again, recapping, putting strategies into effect – a whole range of mental skills that we take for granted but which allow us to have a great deal of control over our lives.

Understanding a situation can be an enormous help in coping with it. Listening carefully to the neuropsychologist's explanations of your loved one's difficulties will go a long way to your being able to handle those difficulties better in the future. Many of the behaviours that result from brain damage can become intensely irritating to other people. In the early weeks and months of the injury sympathy and sorrow are likely to be the emotional lenses through which you view everything. It may be hard for you at this point to realize that some of your loved one's difficulties could ever be irritating. But with the passing of time, life will return to some sort of normality and once again you will have separate strands to your lives. Your waking thoughts will no longer be fully occupied by this trauma or illness. You will be subject to other pressures, other stresses, and it is when you are struggling to cope with these that the invisible disabilities of brain injury can be so intensely infuriating. *You* need to hurry through the early morning routine in order to meet a tight deadline, but your loved one must go through things in precisely the same, plodding order. *Your* mind is preoccupied with today's big meeting and you could do with running through the schedule one more time as you drive your wife to the day centre; but you can't manage that *and* the answering of the same daily string of predictable questions.

There will always be times when stressful circumstances or simple mood will affect your ability to cope with brain injury. But it does help to try and keep in mind the reasons for your loved one's apparent unreasonableness, such as your wife's inability to be flexible with the early morning routine. Again, if you can make an effort to understand why she needs to ask the same questions over and over again, or to know what it is that has robbed her of her memory, you do at least have rational explanations to help you calm your irritation and try to persuade yourself into a more patient response.

In addition to simply explaining the particular difficulties the brain injured individual is experiencing, the neuropsychologist may also be able to make use of particular exercises in thinking to help your loved one use what ability they have to the best effect. They might also be able to suggest strategies towards overcoming particularly problematic areas of behaviour so that, over time, changes may take place and perhaps more independence be regained.

Referral to a *neuropsychiatrist* may also be made at some stage. Sometimes there can be psychiatric complications from brain injury, for example depression, hallucinations (seeing or hearing things that aren't actually present), and confabulation (see page 6). In itself, the fact of having experienced a brain injury and the associated needs to adjust to a new self, a new life and various losses can lead to a clinical depression. If the injury was the result of a road traffic accident or a fall from a height, the shock of the event may result in a post-traumatic stress disorder.

## *Consultations*

The dividing line between these different disciplines is not always clear. Indeed it seems to be becoming more blurred as the knowledge and understanding of brain function increases, thanks to research going on within the various different academic disciplines. Specialists from different backgrounds and training – the neurologist, psychologist, and psychiatrist – may end up with an interest in and experience of dealing with the same sort of conditions. The difference between them may well lie simply in 'where they are coming from' – the sort of angle they take on the condition and how it should be treated. So a range of people with similar problems resulting from brain injury may end up seeing specialists in differently named disciplines. Sometimes the choice of who to refer to may be decided by your GP's or consultant's personal acquaintance with one particular specialist, or on their knowledge of and respect for that specialist's work.

You are likely to approach each of these consultations with a sense of hope, looking forward to some help, some further improvement, and some positive ideas towards enhancing the situation the two of you are in. But understanding of the brain is still limited, and it may well turn out that there is little apparent result from the consultation, and all after a substantial investment on your part. For one thing, the time and energy needed to get your loved one there are likely to be considerable, given the nature of their difficulty. You will have had to organize the practicalities of what might be a journey of some distance and explain everything to your partner, quite likely several times over. You may have had to take time off work, arrange childcare, cajole and encourage your partner to come along with you and struggle through public transport systems or traffic under the stress of possible anger outbursts, persistent questioning or challenging behaviour. Then, after negotiating a maze of hospital corridors, when you finally arrive at the appointment, you will no doubt be asked to recount the whole story of the brain injury again. This in itself is stressful when you have to relive the pain of loss, of trauma, of hurt. And what is the outcome? Perhaps someone does have a good idea of what to do, a new treatment that can be tried, or news of some new research. But perhaps your hopes are dashed, and this latest expert can offer nothing further.

Whatever ideas are forthcoming, whether big, small or nonexistent, there is at least one thing to hang on to. You have done your best. Whenever it is that you begin to accept what has happened, to accept that this is how it is now, that there is no further medical intervention to be made, you will at least know that you have left no stone unturned for the sake of your shared future. And that is a very important piece of knowledge. So take these referrals as a step along the way, even if you think it unlikely to be worth all the effort involved. Try to be thankful that someone is doing their utmost for you both. That effort may well be rewarded. Don't give up hope – but try not to hope extravagantly.

## Other professionals

If you are lucky, the *counsellor* will be an important member of the team in the rehabilitation setting. Rehabilitation is defined as the restoration of a newly disabled person to the best possible degree of normal life. That is clearly going to involve their psychological adjustment to what has happened to them, which is likely to need a lot of talking through. But it is not only the injured person who needs to adjust, and the counsellor on the staff of a rehabilitation centre is generally available to meet with other members of the family too.

If there is no counsellor available, an outside referral is always possible, for whichever member of the family; for the inpatient via the ward sister or charge nurse; for other members of the family via the GP. But it needs to be said that there may well be a long wait to see someone under the National Health Service as there is a great demand for counselling services. Private counselling can be found much more quickly, but at a cost. And do take care to check qualifications and seek references to be sure that what you are paying for is worth having.

Another source of 'listening' help is the *chaplaincy* service. Chaplains from a variety of faiths will be available to patients. All hospitals have full-time or part-time chaplains, and if the rehabilitation centre does not actually have a chaplain on the staff, there will be someone available if you ask. A chaplain may or may, not visit as a matter of course, but they will be only too pleased to respond to a request to meet. Chaplains are very experienced in dealing with people going through situations of deep distress and will offer a non-judgemental listening ear, as well as prayer if that is what you would like. They will be guided by your wishes, and certainly not seek to impose faith on you but to offer what comfort and consolation they can.

If the brain injury is serious, a referral is likely to be made to the hospital social worker. There will be a lot of issues for you to face at some stage, to do with work, housing and finances. It can all seem overwhelming but the social worker is there to help you. They will proceed with caution, a step at a time, giving you space to take things on board and come to terms gradually with the unfolding circumstances of change. They will be acquainted with current regulations in terms of employment, and will know about benefits entitlement and all the ins and outs of when and how these must be claimed. They will, but only if you wish, act as an intermediary between your loved one (and yourself if you are having to act for them) and their employer; between yourselves and any landlord, and between yourselves and the benefits office, if necessary. They may also be able to offer some temporary assistance with things like the costs of hospital visiting, reduced charges for parking during a long-term stay in hospital, and the provision of hospital transport for your loved one to make a visit home if that is possible.

A recent development in the National Health Service is the provision of the *Patient Advice and Liaison Service*. Every healthcare trust now has a 'PALS' – a department which is there to act independently to sort out *your* concerns; that is, the concerns of any patient and/or patient's family regarding their treatment by the health service. They can provide you with full information about NHS services that exist both locally and nationally. It is also their role to liaise with staff and managers in the health service – and where appropriate, other organizations too – to negotiate solutions to difficulties and bring about changes in the way that services are delivered so as to improve quality of care. They can also refer patients or their families to specific local or national support agencies.

Of course, more often than not, the hospital staff, or staff at your local health centre, are able to give you the information you require, make referrals on, or respond to your concerns. But sometimes you may feel wary of raising concerns with the staff on whom you are depending so closely. And certainly if your concerns are resolving themselves into a complaint you can feel very vulnerable and anxious that you might be putting the ongoing care of your loved one at risk because of bad feeling. This fear should be unfounded; the medical staff are professionals, with a duty to care properly for everyone, whatever personal feelings may come into play. But when you are going through a period of intense emotion the ground beneath you can feel very unstable. It may well feel a lot safer to have a third party available to act independently – and unemotion-ally – on your behalf.

The *case manager* generally comes into play only in situations where there has been an award of damages. In terms of brain injury, this is going to relate only to traumatic injury or perhaps anoxia, caused by someone's negligence or criminal action, when a court case has been brought and won. When substantial damages are awarded because of severe and lasting disability and dependence, a case manager may be employed to organize and manage the injured person's ongoing care and rehabilitation. They may arrange suitable accommodation, seeing to its adaptation as necessary; interview, appoint and manage a team of care workers; arrange sessions with therapists as appropriate; organize a routine of daily or weekly activities; claim benefits and manage the budget; and generally act as attorney and advocate for the individual concerned. Case managers are mostly self-employed, often with a background in social work. It should go without saying that qualifications, references and track records need to be thoroughly checked before a case manager is appointed. Those with power of attorney can make the appointment, usually a member of the immediate family, or possibly the lawyer representing the victim to whom the damages have been awarded.

A last but key professional in the whole string of them will be *your GP*. If your crisis is the result of illness, the GP's surgery is likely to have been the place where the whole thing started. If it started in the accident and emergency department, your GP will have been informed of the admission by the hospital.

Relationships with GPs vary enormously. GPs vary. Their patients vary. It is a two-way relationship that works best when it is founded on trust. Let's hope that your relationship is a good one as – if the brain injury is severe – your family doctor is likely to be a mainstay in the life of your family over the next few years.

The GP acts as gatekeeper to much of the healthcare provided by the NHS and, once the patient has been discharged from the hospital service, any further help in terms of ongoing medical or therapeutic care on the NHS will need to be sought via the GP. So it is worth trying hard to keep – or to put – that relationship on a right footing. This can be difficult if you feel that, for whatever reason, the GP is stopping you from having what you want. No doubt she has good reason for this, and if you are to trust her, she will need to be prepared to explain this to you. Similarly, if she is to trust your opinion and recognize your concerns as genuine and not based on fantasy, you will need to be able to explain these clearly to her, and be ready to back them up with as much evidence as possible.

Those who are articulate and assertive have a much better chance of negotiating our welfare systems successfully. If you are not a good communicator (and you may well not be at present because of your close emotional involvement in a very stressful situation), don't hesitate to ask someone else to come along and put your case to the GP for you. If that isn't possible, spend some time before your consultation on your own, or better still with a friend, writing down everything you want to say. Don't be afraid to refer to this in the surgery, or even to hand it to your GP if that is easiest for you. Any doctor worth their salt will have some understanding of what you are going through, and will be keen to make the consultation as manageable for you as possible.

Your doctor has a duty to provide care for all the family, and will be able to take a more objective view of the situation than you can. You may not like their views of the way forward, but don't dismiss what is said out of hand; try to take time to consider the doctor's comments thoughtfully. Unfortunately, many patient–doctor relationships break down at times of severe stress, and often because the close carer cannot accept that the doctor is working on their behalf, that the doctor wants as much as they do to see the best possible outcome. Or that, where there has been a mistake made, or where care has been less than perfect, nothing will be gained by a tightly held grudge. If the two of you can work together, with mutual respect, it will be best for all concerned.

# 5

## What can *I* do?

### *Loving, caring, talking*

In the early days, it may well seem that all you can do is get from one day to the next. You will learn how to 'take one day at a time'. You may wonder what the future may bring, but there is no energy to spare in worrying about it. There will be no time to dwell on the past. Your major concern will be in the present with the progress of your loved one, managing the practical necessities of daily life at the same time.

Anchor yourself as firmly as you can in the present. You can invest the present in your future together, by putting your efforts as much as possible into the patient's care. You may not have the expertise of the professionals, but you do have something extremely valuable to offer. In a word, love. There is good evidence to show that, in the field of brain injury, individuals who are surrounded by a loving family make a much better recovery than those who are struggling on their own.

You know this patient like none of the professionals can. Your loving touch, your loving voice are much more closely tuned in to their mind and body than anyone else's, and therefore far more likely to break through any barriers to communication. Even if the patient is in a coma, it is still a good idea to talk to them. Encourage them by pointing out to them any little bits of progress they've made, let them know what's happening in the world, what the family's up to, pass on messages from friends, and tell them you love them.

It's thought that hearing is the last of the senses to stop functioning as levels of consciousness drop, and there have been remarkable stories of apparently deeply unconscious people who have still heard what was said around them and known what was going on. You may feel awkward and embarrassed at first, holding a one-sided conversation in the midst of the intensive care unit (ICU), but you will soon overcome this once you make a start and get into the swing of it. And the risk of missing the chance of better progress by not talking is just too great to take.

Loving and caring also mean that you get stuck in there, and do your very best to work with the professionals for your loved one's best recovery. Depending on your work situation of course, it might be the case that you are able to spend more hours at this particular bedside than a therapist who has perhaps 15 or 20 others on her case list. Under guidance from the physiotherapist, you can help exercise muscles to stop them wasting. You can help desensitize the mouth according to the speech therapist's instructions. Always check with the therapist concerned, but the likelihood is that the more times such exercises are carried out the better.

And you must now be your loved one's advocate. If you used to be the shy, retiring type, you may have to change for a few months. At the moment your loved one is unable to fight their own corner. It's up to you now to do that. It's not about fighting against any person, but fighting with the rest of the team against brain damage. Try to keep alert to what is going on. Ask all the questions you can – don't let a fear of appearing foolish stop some important information from reaching you. Be ready to offer information about your loved one's past or personality that may have a bearing on the situation. And if it should happen that you think some of the treatment or care is not being carried out as it should be, it will be up to you to point this out.

Equally though, if you are someone who flies off the handle when things go wrong, try to be aware that this sort of behaviour is rarely constructive. Don't fall into the trap of letting your anger about what has happened fall onto the doctors or other professionals. That way only bitterness lies. Try to curb your temper and aim to be gently but firmly assertive to make sure that team members pull their weight and explain things clearly to you. Try to point out sympathetically (we all know how hard pressed hospital staff are) if something has been left undone. If you think something has been mismanaged, drawing attention to it with a slightly mystified question should mean that it will be put right at the earliest opportunity, without antagonizing anyone in the process. You are – or should be – an important and valued member of the team working for your loved one's best future. Play your own part to the best of your ability.

Yes, this is a counsel of perfection. But it really is worth bringing all your best team-playing ability into the hospital situation. If you need to let off steam after being the model of good temper in the face of a serious oversight, or shrink to a shaking jelly after standing up to a bossy and powerful member of staff, do it at home among friends or family. They are there to support you and will understand.

## *Staying positive*

It seems to be true in life that those who believe they will be successful are successful. There's a lot to be said for staying positive, but it doesn't mean that you have to be a paragon of strength and intelligence all the time. In fact, it's probably healthier for you if you're not! It would be a strange thing indeed if you didn't feel or express any upset over what has happened. This is a brain injury that your loved one has suffered – and in a very real sense, because this sort of injury is bound to affect the relationship between you, you have suffered it too.

You are likely to feel overwhelmed at times. You need to take in the reality of what has happened in order to adjust to a new situation. How can you begin to adjust unless you admit to your grief, your shock, your upset? If you let your grief out when you can do so safely, the chances are you will be able to bounce back. Yes, you will have your very low and very tearful times. Having these – and having them in their rightful place, in the privacy of your own home and family – might well allow you to be strong at the bedside for your loved one's sake, and strong in conversation with the professionals. No member of staff will mind if you get emotional at times, but a complete loss of control does tend to get in the way of communication.

Staying positive does not mean that you have to pretend that everything is bright and rosy. What it does mean is that you refuse to take a failure as a defeat. If something hasn't worked today, keep trying because it might work tomorrow. If it hasn't worked after lots and lots of tomorrows, then it's still not time to give up, but it may be time to look for another way, for something else to try. And it's important to take stock of progress that has been made. Try looking at the situation through the eyes of a less frequent visitor; they will notice the changes and the progress far more readily than you who are living in its midst.

Don't forget to give yourself credit for all your efforts and what they have contributed towards this progress. If, today, you are finding it all hard going and have let something slip, don't blame yourself. Focus instead on what you have managed. Remind yourself that nobody's perfect, that's it's understandable if you are working at less than your best; you are under a lot of pressure. Allow yourself the break that you need in the understanding that it will make for better efforts again when you are rested.

You are, after all, getting stuck in for a long haul. The time in hospital may be a couple of weeks. It may stretch into months. After hospital there may be a stay in a rehabilitation unit, for at least one month, more likely several, even possibly a year or more. Even after that longed-for day when your loved one returns home, life will not be as it was before. Perhaps most difficult of all is the fact that in the early days no one will be able to predict what sort of recovery might be made.

You will need resources to sustain you in this long haul. Friends to ease some of the pain, share in your grief, listen to your worries – and sometimes to take you out of your situation and remind you that other things are going on in the world. It may even be helpful to take up an activity which will drive everything else out of your mind from time to time and give you something else to focus on. This might be a good time for some piano lessons, for example, or to learn some yoga, or take up running. Take care of yourself; you are giving a lot out, and need to make sure you put something back in.

## Coping with fear

In this long haul, you may well be very afraid. Will I be able to cope? Am I coping? What will my loved one be like? Will we have to move house? Will we have enough money? Will we have any friends? Will I still be able to love him or her? What if I too get ill? Your fear may be any or all of these, or others still. Or it may be unspecific, without any particular shape or form, just one great big ball of fear.

Try to pin down what it is that you're afraid of. A fear that is named is much easier to conquer, because you can then start lining up against it armies of reason and experience. For example, a very common fear might be whether there will be enough money. If the fear isn't faced it will continue to haunt you. If you turn and look at it rationally you can argue with it. 'We've been hard up before and managed – if we have to cut down we will.' 'Awful things have happened to other people I know and they've lost their jobs – but they still manage.' 'We've got a good family around us – they won't see us go under.' 'Things change, life moves on – I might get a better-paid job in a couple of years' time.' And so on. The fear already seems smaller, less powerful.

It may be that your own fear is bigger than that one. It may be that the source of your fear is that a life which seemed predictable, secure, known and understood, has quite out of the blue turned upside down with all your previous certainties scattered to the four winds. This is a very powerful fear. But whatever the fear, however powerful, naming it brings it down to size. Even this fear, once its form is recognized and its limits are named, can be argued with. 'Yes, life has turned upside down. But it will settle again. It might take on a new shape, but it will have its own certainties once more. This storm will come to an end in due time.' 'Other people have gone through times like these. They have survived. They are often stronger as a result. I too will survive.' 'Just because my life has turned upside down at the moment, there is no reason to suppose everything is unpredictable. This has happened now, and it is not likely to happen again. I can still move forward with confidence.'

Of course, such arguments with yourself will be ongoing ones over a period of time. Fears are not so easily dismissed. So once you have recognized that you are afraid, be ready to talk seriously to the fears, reminding yourself over and over of the arguments against them. Speak compassionately with yourself, though. It's not stupid to be afraid. It makes perfect sense. But it's not necessarily very helpful. Fear can be crippling.

Sharing your fears, talking them through, whether with a trusted friend or with a professional counsellor, can also be a big help. There's something about bringing them into the open, putting them into speech and outside of you, that in itself reduces their power and brings them down to size. An added bonus is that the person you talk to may well be able to contribute their own reasons and experience to serve as allies to yours and increase the likelihood of conquering that particular fear once and for all.

## *Looking after yourself*

Looking after yourself more generally is important too. A lot of demands are being made on you both physically and emotionally just now, and it's important for both you and your loved one that you are able to meet those demands. The time and energy taken up with hospital visiting, running a home, perhaps a job and a family too, will no doubt make it extra difficult, but try all you can to keep up a balanced diet and to get enough sleep. You may have to take your sleep in snatches, on the bus or train, or even at the hospital bedside – but try to get it by hook or by crook.

It may be difficult for practical reasons for you to take a break from the situation, but if the opportunity arises, do all you can to take it. The hardest thing at the moment may be to make the emotional separation necessary to allow you to go away, but remember you are not being selfish in looking after yourself.

A break does not have to be long for it to be refreshing. Yes, a week by the sea might be what is really needed, but even a day's walking in the hills, half a day in an art gallery, an evening at a concert, or just half an hour sitting in the park enjoying the birds and flowers can all work wonders. Rather than just slumping down in front of some mindless TV, try to take breaks that will feed your spirit and give you something to draw on in the tougher moments.

## *Looking ahead (with care)*

Eventually the time will come when you are safe to look ahead. There is going to be a future! And its shape – at least for the next year or so – has at last become clearer. So look ahead you must, even though now, having gradually learned to take things one day at a time, you may find it difficult. There will be plans to make, adjustments both mental and practical to carry through, and no doubt an extraordinary amount of patience required. It is no easy thing discharging someone from hospital with ongoing needs to be met. There may well be a time lapse of a week or several before a discharge that has been talked about turns into a reality. It will be important to ensure that continuing care is in place, whether the patient is moving home or to a rehabilitation unit.

It is vital that you are honest now about any feelings you might have about the move. If your loved one is being discharged home, things should move at a pace that gives you time to prepare both in practical terms and emotionally for what might well be a huge undertaking and a fearfully big responsibility. If your loved one remains very disabled (physically, mentally or both) there should be a graduated discharge to ease the situation – a few hours before whole days at home, then an overnight stay, a whole weekend, and so on. If it becomes too much at any stage you must feel able to say – you would be doing neither yourself nor your loved one any favours if you pretend you are ready before you actually are.

In addition you will need to have your own support structures in place before the discharge. Make sure your family and friends are aware of what you are doing. Their care and concern will help support you emotionally, while a relief care worker coming in on a regular basis to make sure you get a break will allow for some physical refreshment. You may well also need to have arrangements for respite care in place, and in many rehabilitation settings it is customary for the bed to be kept open for a couple of weeks after discharge in case things don't work out. Try to set a pace for the arrangements that you feel comfortable with. There's no shame in taking things slowly, or admitting you can't handle the situation. The real shame would be in pretending you can and destroying the welfare of yourself and those around you that you love.

Yes, you need to be looking ahead as this stage comes upon you, but look ahead with care. On the one hand, look into the immediate future in some detail and with serious thought. On the other hand, don't be looking ahead to the whole of the rest of your lives and imagining it is all laid out for you. No one can know for sure what the future holds. Nothing is set in stone. For now, this is how it is. For the next week, month or so, this is how it is likely to be. And for now, that's enough. Leave it at that.

# 6

## *What if?* A range of possible outcomes

The shock of your loved one's brain injury can make *you* feel very disconnected from the real world. Depending on how much of yourself was invested in this particular relationship, you may feel that, having lost their real presence, conversation, comments and reactions to what you do and say, you have also lost sight of yourself. Life might take on a dream-like existence; people comment that they feel as though they are living in a film, watching themselves going through the motions of life. The temptation then is to expect the film to come to an end, your partner to come home from hospital and life to resume just as it was before. Unfortunately, that's not how it works.

With an injury to the brain as with an injury to no other part of the body, there is a vast range of possible outcomes. Just as each and every brain is individual, reflecting a unique personality with its own particular abilities, preferences, thought processes, moods, insights, sense of humour, and so on, so each and every brain injury is individual. No one person will be left with precisely the same difficulties as any one other.

But that said, this vast range of possible outcomes can be broken down according to the level of remaining difficulty, whether physical or mental, or a combination of both. There will be people with differing problems, but who require a similar amount of care within a certain type of care setting, depending on the severity of the injury that has occurred and the amount of recovery that has followed.

There is a usual sequence of care after a serious brain injury. The injured person will first be admitted to hospital; there might be an initial period in the intensive care ward, followed, when things are more stable, by a period of treatment in an 'ordinary' ward. This might be a surgical, medical or neurological ward, depending on the type of injury (and whether or not the hospital concerned has a neurological ward). As recovery progresses and the body's own healing systems have had time to do their stuff, the injured person is likely to be moved to a rehabilitation setting. This may itself be a ward within a hospital, or it may be a designated residential rehabilitation centre. It may offer rehabilitation to people who have suffered all sorts of injuries or it may exist solely for those who have suffered a brain injury. After a period of time here, the brain injured person might return to living at home.

But this sequence of care can stick at any point, depending on the brain's capacity to heal itself, and/or on its response to treatment and to rehabilitation. We have already mentioned *persistent vegetative state*, in which the injured person remains in a trance-like state, unable to be aroused, with very little if any control over their body. This person, unable to turn themselves in a bed, and most likely without control over bladder or bowels, will need continuous nursing care in a hospital setting.

Assuming that the injured person does emerge from coma, the body will need a period of rest and recuperation during which to follow its natural process of recovery, for swelling to subside, for wounds to heal and tissues and cells to mend themselves after trauma. But even after time allowed for this, the injured person will not be the same as their former self, and, in order to maximize their recovery, rehabilitation will be necessary.

## Rehabilitation

Rehabilitation is the restoration of a disabled person to some degree of normal life through appropriate training. Muscles will have become wasted and weak during the considerable period of bedrest, and the trauma to the brain will have caused it to lose much of its ability to control the body. The appropriate training will involve working muscles not only to strengthen them but also to re-educate the brain to regain control. For example, the brain injured person may well need to learn how to walk again. The physiotherapist will help with this by guiding the body through the necessary movements. This not only feeds back information to the brain as to what it needs to instruct the body to do, but also strengthens the wasted muscles so that in due course they can carry out independently the actions that the brain has relearned to order from them.

The patient's level of ability in a range of *activities of daily living* will be assessed over the first few weeks after admission to a rehabilitation unit. These activities include such things as getting dressed, washing in a shower or bath, washing hair, making a cup of tea or a light snack, climbing stairs, using a knife and fork, and so on.

During the rehabilitation process a team of therapists will work at these activities with the patient, and the ability to carry out the activities will be regularly reassessed in order to measure objectively any progress being made. It may be that a level of ability will be reached in every activity that makes it possible for the individual to return to living independently at home, if necessary with various pieces of adaptive equipment in place. But, again, progress may become stuck at any stage, for either physical or mental reasons, or a combination of both. For example, the individual may not be able to regain the strength and control to be able to move themselves safely from a bed to a chair. Or perhaps they are unable to sequence properly the necessary actions involved in making a hot drink. Memory or awareness may be so severely damaged that it would not be safe for this person to be left alone in a kitchen with a gas cooker.

If it proves impossible for the person to be rehabilitated enough to return to living at home independently, they may perhaps be able to return to living at home with others present to help them through the day and/or night as necessary. These others may be members of family or friends, but it should be stressed that social services are not allowed to assume that a married partner, a parent or other close family member will take responsibility for care. In the absence of family to provide care, the ongoing care needs must be provided for by social services. Whether this care can be provided in the home setting will depend on the amount necessary in any individual case. Home care workers may be used to 'top up' a basis of care or supervision provided by family, but the cost of this provision means that social services as a general rule set an upper limit on the number of hours of home care per week they will provide.

## *Residential care*

So what if someone can't return to living at home? If rehabilitation sticks at a point where independent living is impossible, or if family members are unable or unwilling to provide the basis of care and supervision necessary for safety, then residential care will have to continue in some form. This may need to be in a nursing home or a simple residential care home, depending on the level of disability that remains.

Another option, depending on what is available in your locality, may be a residential unit attached to a rehabilitation centre. Such units allow people to be given a level of simple supervision and assistance, but also to continue to receive over a longer period of time some rehabilitative training towards becoming more independent and engaging in meaningful activities and a fulfilling social life.

Although a period of two or three years is often quoted as the length of time after which no further recovery of the brain will take place, there are experts who consider that recovery continues right up until the end of life. The brain heals at a very slow pace. It also has a capacity to adapt itself to new situations, albeit, again, at a snail's pace. It would therefore seem that, second only perhaps to returning to live at home among a caring and supportive family, the best option would be a designated brain injury centre, where stimulation and strategies are devised and maintained with a view to ongoing improvement, at whatever rate.

Nowadays there are also some smaller residential units to be found, specifically managed for people with brain injuries. Sometimes these are purpose-built units that cater for the whole range of physical disabilities. But some take the form of an ordinary house in an ordinary street, shared by four to six brain injured individuals who may seem to be more or less independent and very able, but actually require oversight and support from someone with understanding of their limitations and difficulties. There will be room on the premises for a care worker to sleep, and other assistants are likely to come daily to help with household and social activities as necessary.

## Home care

A growing number of healthcare trusts now employ a team of workers dedicated to the *structured community rehabilitation* of the brain injured. In this case, after a certain amount of progress has been made, the patient will be discharged from the rehabilitation centre, and therapists and rehabilitation assistants from the community team will visit the home to help with further rehabilitation. This would seem to be a better way forward than an extended residential stay. For one thing, rehabilitation can be precisely geared to the individual's normal environment instead of to the rather artificial setting of the hospital or rehabilitation centre. And in addition, the individual's emotional state is likely to be that much better for being in their own home that their receptiveness to further training is likely to be at its best.

At some stage there will come a point where the therapists involved agree that no more significant rehabilitation is likely and they will withdraw their services. From this point onwards, any ongoing care and support that are needed in the home, if not provided by family, are likely to be provided by home care workers, through an agency to whom social services contract out. These workers have a very basic level of training in care work but are usually without any specific qualifications. They can be wonderful; they can be barely capable. The problem is that you generally have to put up with whoever is sent.

Since April 2003 all local councils have been required to make *direct payments* available to all disabled people who are eligible, i.e. 'willing and able' to manage the payments. Under this scheme, disabled people can recruit and employ their own care workers and assistants. They have to set up a separate personal bank account into which the money to which they are entitled for social services care is paid according to their assessed need. From this fund they then pay employees' wages or, if they prefer – and can afford – to use an agency, the agency bills. The disabled individual decides where to advertise for staff, writes their own job description and person specification (with help if they need it) and, hopefully, finds people who share their own attitudes to life, so they feel comfortable with them and happy to have them working in their home. The downside is the considerable responsibility involved in becoming an employer, which is why the brain injured individual may well need some other family member to be acting on their behalf in this respect.

Whether the person concerned is using direct payments or ordinary social services provision, the responsibility always rests with social services to carry out a *needs assessment*. The current and ongoing needs of the disabled person will be set down according to reports from specialist staff who have been involved in their care so far. The injured person and family members will also have the opportunity to contribute to this, and to argue with the assessment made. But once this assessment is finalized and agreed by all concerned, social services must draw up a *care plan* that will serve to meet those needs. They then have a legal obligation to allocate the necessary funds and ensure that those needs are met. The care plan will have to be reviewed regularly, on an annual basis at least, though usually more often than this at first, in case there should be a change of circumstance involving either an increase or decrease in the amount of care needed.

Each stage of the caring sequence during the recovery process, and each one of these possible outcomes, will involve both a mental and a physical adjustment and a coming to terms, both for the injured person and for you. As you reach the high of progressing to the next stage of recovery only to hit the doldrums of slow months of repetitive strategies, or the anxiety of whether another landmark will be reached, amid the fatigue of all that you are having to manage in the meantime, you do indeed seem to be riding that now proverbial emotional roller coaster.

## Are you to be the carer?

In the midst of all that, you will need to consider carefully how much you want to be involved in the whole process, and how much responsibility you want to assume for ongoing care. There may be no question in your mind that you want to get stuck in and help full-time. There may be no possibility of your doing this because of responsibilities for other members of the family, because of financial demands that force you to remain in employment, or because you would, quite honestly, find more frustration than satisfaction in that sort of lifestyle. You will need to try to take a long, hard, cold look at the situation, weighing up all the various possibilities. Talk extensively about these with other members of the family and with your friends, listening hard to their comments, whether they fall in line with your current way of thinking or not. Consider the effect of the decision you make on other members of the family; do they need to be given some say in it? If so, what practical help and support would they offer in which circumstances?

Take a long, cold, hard look at yourself too and whether you are cut out for the life of a carer. Try to separate off the pity you feel around this dreadful thing happening to the person you love so much, and consider whether you could cope with being in the company of someone with these particular disabilities for the bulk of your time. Perhaps the disabilities would make for a physically hard day; are you up to it? Perhaps they would require unlimited reserves of patience and tolerance; do you have them? Perhaps you are making light of the disabilities and the difficulties of living with them full-time because they are invisible. Sometimes these are the hardest to cope with. The very fact that they are invisible makes them difficult to get hold of, which in turn makes it hard for us to credit ourselves with tolerance or patience because there seems to be little there to be patient or tolerant with. On top of which there may be little in the way of support or sympathy from people outside of the situation because they can't see the difficulties either – which adds to your confusion as to what precisely the difficulties are.

Talk also to the social worker. She can't make your decision for you, but she will have some helpful information to offer. She may be able to give examples (anonymous) of how other people have managed a similar situation to yours. She will be able to tell you what sort of back-up you would get as a carer. What sort of help would you get to give you a break during the week, and how often? Respite care should be available, but what is the local provision? Is it suitable? How much would you qualify for?

As if the emotional and practical sides of things aren't enough, there are also financial implications to your decision. Residential care – whether ongoing or on a respite basis – needs to be paid for, and contributions towards this have to be means-tested. If the two of you have been sharing income you will need to work out whether you alone can manage household finances with a very much reduced contribution from your partner. The bulk of their income, if any, is likely to go towards their care, though there will be allowance made for family responsibilities. Social services levy a charge for home care services; this varies from district to district, and the highest contribution is generally way below the actual cost of the service provided, but can nevertheless be a considerable drain on the budget. Could you manage without going to work yourself? What benefits would you be eligible for? Would they be sufficient? The social worker will be able to provide you with the facts and figures about benefits and charges, but only you will be able to make the final decision about managing financially in a particular set of circumstances.

In the case of a traumatic brain injury there may well be one other big financial consideration. If the injury was caused by a road traffic accident, or by assault, or by someone else's negligence, it may be possible to sue for compensation. Numerous legal firms now specialize in cases such as these and you will have seen many advertisements relating to 'no win, no fee' compensation cases. Indeed, if the accident your partner was involved in appeared in the local news, one or more such firms may well have approached you to tout for business.

Tread carefully. There are many unscrupulous firms out there, and it would be wise to consider their motives. In any case, you should ponder the matter thoroughly and take plenty of advice from as many sources as possible among your friends, family and acquaintances – perhaps even from the Citizens' Advice Bureau – before embarking on any lawsuit. Rage at what has happened is totally understandable, but it may be worthwhile taking time to talk about what has happened, and to obtain plenty of feedback, before rushing into litigation in haste out of – possibly misplaced – anger at your loved one's misfortune. You will need to weigh up the energies it will require of you – which may well be better invested elsewhere. Take into account the likely length of such a process, the emotional costs to you, and the potential financial needs of the injured person. These will all need to be carefully balanced, remembering that any large amount of compensation won may well make this other decision about ongoing care an awful lot easier, offering the possibility of employing a case manager to handle ongoing care arrangements within the home, leaving you free to follow an independent lifestyle.

But whatever you decide about how much to involve yourself in the care and rehabilitation of your loved one, the important thing to remember is this: this is the way you are doing things today. Tomorrow it might change. In the first weeks and months you will in any case be feeling your way – getting to know and learning to accommodate this new person in your life, muddling through with the household budget, coming to terms with what has happened and how it has impacted on you. There should be others alongside you supporting you in this: the social worker, the GP, any medical or therapeutic staff still involved, a counsellor perhaps, and your family and close friends. In the early days, if you realize you have made a wrong decision, that you are not handling the situation well, that you need more help than you thought you would, or that you need to get away from it all, these others – especially the professionals – should be able to move fairly quickly to relieve the situation. But at every stage along the way you remain a free individual. Don't let others judge you for your decision, and don't let yourself feel trapped by it. Make it for now, not for ever.

# 7

## Practical adjustments

### *Living arrangements*

A homecoming won't happen all at once. There will have been visits beforehand, first of all with one or more professionals in tow. The occupational therapist (usually from the local social services department, although sometimes from the hospital) will need to view the set-up at home, whether your living arrangements will be accessible and safe, bearing in mind the particular circumstances of the acquired disability. If your loved one is able to walk, it may be a simple case of handrails where there are steps or grabrails to help with getting in and out of the bath. If eyesight has been affected, improved lighting might be necessary, or adjustments may need to be made to the heating system or electrics to make them safely manageable. If only simple adaptations are needed, the therapist can usually set things in motion quickly, and under a certain limit – currently £250 to £500 depending upon the local authority – these will be paid for by the department.

Sometimes though, adaptations need to be more extreme. If for example your loved one is now confined to a wheelchair, doors may need widening and ramps fitting to allow for access into the house or into all its various rooms. A stairlift may be needed, or even an extension downstairs to accommodate a bathroom and bedroom on one level with the living room and kitchen. Worktops, cupboards and sink may need lowering.

In such circumstances as these you will be offered a financial assessment. You may qualify for a disabled facilities grant. Works that qualify for a grant need to be 'necessary, appropriate, reasonable and practicable'. And so the likelihood of your getting a grant will depend not only on the level of disability but also the type and age of the property. Councils are not likely to pay out huge sums to adapt a property when it might actually make much better financial – and practical – sense for you to move home.

This possibility may need to be faced. There are several reasons why you may need or want to consider moving house now. You may need to move for the sake of more practical accommodation as described; it may be that purpose-built accommodation for the disabled, provided by a housing association perhaps, would be the ideal solution for you now. You may need to move because the brain injury has lost your loved one his job; perhaps your accommodation was provided as part of that job, or perhaps the loss of income means you can no longer afford to live where you lived before.

Moving house is known to be one of the most stressful events in a lifetime. But given your present circumstances, it may be put into a different perspective, that of just one more thing that needs sorting out. The most stressful thing will be if you need to find accommodation at short notice. If you are renting from the council, or if you are falling behind with mortgage payments, there are usually systems in place to make allowances, or to restructure payments, for periods of extreme illness and life changes. They are likely to be sympathetic, but it is up to you to let them know what is happening, and you are probably well advised to put them in the picture at the first hint of the possibility that you might need special treatment. This applies to a private landlord too, though they may not have the means to make such long-term allowances for your difficulties.

The most draconian of housing arrangements in the UK is tied accommodation, where a home is linked in with someone's employment. If your loved one has been working in the licensing trade for example, or as a farm labourer, a minister of religion, a teacher in a private school – any number of jobs – your housing may well have been provided as part of the working package. If the work required can no longer be carried out, that housing will be needed for the replacement in post. If this is your situation, you may well not have much notice to leave.

You may be fortunate enough to have a sympathetic landlord, willing to extend that period of notice for as long as possible, understanding the difficulties that you are in. But it may be that you need to act quickly. Enlist the help of the hospital social worker, who should be able to make it their business to find out your rights in this situation. If these rights are not sufficient to give you the necessary security, at least to allow for a breathing space, they should then be able to get in touch with the council and argue the priority of your need for housing.

This may be a good time to find out about any welfare services that might be tied in with your loved one's employment. If your loved one belongs to a trade union or professional association, they may well be able to offer help. Most if not all unions offer legal representation and advice, which may be useful if you are considering a compensation claim in the case of traumatic injury. Many also have benevolent funds or include insurance to assist in just such a situation as this, where sudden disability throws a member's life into confusion. There may also be a welfare officer, whose precise working role can be flexible to the particular needs of their members at any given time. It is certainly worth asking – or asking the hospital social worker to ask on your behalf. If your own life is frantic with hospital visiting, supporting children and other associated pressures, such a welfare officer may be able to put in some of the necessary legwork around disputes over accommodation, finding a new home if necessary, and finding the necessary finance, a mortgage or bridging loan. While they will not, of course, take decisions for you, they can be useful gatherers of information so that you have the right materials to hand in order to be able to make the necessary decisions yourself.

## Driving and transport

A licence-holder is required to notify the Driver and Vehicle Licensing Authority (DVLA) if they suffer a severe head injury, brain surgery, brain tumour, stroke (with any symptoms lasting longer than a month), epilepsy, serious memory problems and/or episodes of confusion (as well as a range of other medical conditions). Given the context of this book, it is likely to be obvious that the injured individual is not fit to drive and you will need to return their driving licence. You can send it with a covering letter outlining the reasons for its return, or you can download a 'declaration of voluntary surrender' from the DVLA's website.

If there is some doubt on your part about fitness to drive, you need to notify the authority of the medical condition and a questionnaire will be sent or, again, you can download the relevant questionnaire from the DVLA's website. Completion of the questionnaire will give the authority more details about the condition of the individual concerned. It will also give the medical advisor to the DVLA permission to request further information from the doctor or specialist involved. As a result of information given, the medical adviser may ask for a further medical examination, or for a driving assessment to be undertaken.

If, as is likely after a severe brain injury, the DVLA decides that your loved one is not fit to drive, the authority will call in the licence. The DVLA must provide a medical explanation for this action and also explain your right of appeal. The authority may give permission for your loved one to reapply for a licence after a certain period of time has passed. Should unimagined improvement take place, your loved one can apply for the licence to be restored, provided they meet the medical standards of fitness to drive. Your GP will be able to advise on this.

Loss of the right to drive may be a severe frustration and the cause of a great deal of tension and anxiety within the household until it is accepted. And unfortunately that can take some time if lack of memory and lack of insight mean that the reasons for not driving have to be pointed out over and over. If someone else in the household drives, keys may need to be carefully hidden. Things might even get to such a pitch that it feels safer just to ignore the car altogether; leave it at a friend's house until its absence is accepted and some adjustment to this limitation made.

The award of the mobility component of the Disability Living Allowance is made specifically for help in getting around (although it does not need to be accounted for). It can be useful for paying ordinary public transport costs or for taxis if the person needs carrying safely from door to door to prevent wandering.

*Motability* is a scheme that has been set up specifically for people in receipt of this benefit, by which they can use this payment towards the cost of purchasing or leasing a car. Normally it applies to disabled people who are themselves able to drive (perhaps with special adaptations to the vehicle), but it can also be used to buy a vehicle for someone else to drive in order to transport the disabled person. You may wish to investigate this scheme further, and contact details are given in 'Useful addresses'.

## Financial adjustments

If the brain injury is severe enough to rob an individual of the ability to run their own affairs, considerable adjustments will need to be made in terms of managing the household finances. However things might have been organized before, the financial management will now fall entirely on your shoulders. If you are married, many bodies will accept your signature on behalf of your spouse. But not all. It may well be best – depending partly on the complexity of your financial circumstances and partly on the particular nature of the brain injury – to take out a *power of attorney*.

You will need to speak to a solicitor about setting this up. You, another member of the family or a friend, can take on a *temporary* power of attorney, which gives you responsibility over someone else's finances and allows you to receive payments on their behalf. The person for whom you are acting will then be able to cancel that power of attorney at any time.

However, if the lawyer involved considers the brain injured person 'mentally incapable' of deciding to appoint and actually appointing a suitable attorney, then an *enduring* power of attorney will need to be registered with the *Court of Protection*. This is a governmental body set up to protect the financial interests of those who are mentally incapable of doing this for themselves. The Court of Protection will appoint a receiver to deal with the individual's day-to-day finances, and any decisions involving your loved one's financial arrangements will be beyond your control.

## Coping with loss of income

This is likely to be quite a frightening time, as you begin to face up to all the implications of your loved one's sudden disability. Whatever the long-term expectations, they are likely to be off work for some time, probably years rather than months. Unless they happen to belong to the small percentage of people who have taken out loss of earnings insurance, their income will be considerably reduced. If you are partners, if you have children, this will have a knock-on effect on you and them. Unfortunately it is always easier to adjust to increased than to reduced income.

On the other hand, it's worth saying that this life-changing event will have given your priorities a really good shake-up. You may well realize now as you have never realized before that the love you hold for the injured person is the bottom line. Hang on to that fact.

Money may well begin to hold less importance for you than it has done in the past, and when its reduced supply is getting to you, you can try reminding yourself of the things that really matter, that you really hold dear.

However, financial worry can be crippling. In our materialistic society it is very easy to place money at the centre of our lives. Then, when its supply feels inadequate, it is as if the engine has seized up and life can't go on.

But remember, however much your income is curtailed, thanks to the welfare state it will be possible to live on what you have. In this country, nobody actually dies from lack of income. You may not be able to live in the way you are accustomed or the way you would like, but you will be able to live. You may have to find different, cheaper sources of pleasure and fun, different and cheaper ways to satisfy your interests and fill your leisure hours – but they are there to be found. They very often need more effort putting in, a determined attitude both to making that extra effort and to finding the pleasure in what might be unorthodox places. But that in itself means they can offer more lasting satisfaction than the sort of pleasure that is handed to you on a plate, that you may enjoy at the time, but which fades quickly from the memory and emotions.

And with the passage of time, when you have been able to adjust to living with disability in the family, if the financial circumstances of your lives are still proving deeply unsatisfactory, there will be steps you can take to improve them. Not every decision must be made now.

## *Dealing with the bank*

Assuming you were in a stable financial situation when the injury occurred, you will have some leeway in which to consider your options before things start to hit home. Of course, you may already have been in some financial difficulty at that point, and you have now been left to carry the can alone. At whatever point the crunch comes, determine not to be afraid. Banks, credit card companies, all institutions that seem 'faceless', are of course made up of human beings with their own life experience. They should not be without understanding if you can explain your circumstances clearly to them. In fact such institutions usually have systems in place by which rules can be bent and payments restructured to cope with just this sort of situation. You may well feel like a completely isolated case, but you are not. Nobody may have presented with exactly your story before, but staff will have come across something similar and they should be sympathetic, or at the very least matter-of-fact. If they are neither of these and their attitude makes you uncomfortable it reflects badly on them, not you; ask to speak to someone else.

It will all be a lot easier – for the bank as well as for you – if you have done your homework beforehand. Try to set down on paper the precise nature of your financial difficulties: how much you owe; what is the shortfall in your monthly income; how much time you will need to sort things out; what monthly payments you can afford, and so on. Try to think of all the questions they might ask, and brainstorm all the possible ways that you can see in which the difficulties could be sorted out. Be ready to explain, quite possibly in some detail, what your precise circumstances and difficulties are. If you are the sort of person whose brain freezes up, or who becomes tongue-tied in a stressful situation, you might want to have everything set out clearly on paper ready to refer to during the crucial conversation.

You may find a face-to-face meeting easier than talking on the phone; the bank (or whatever the company is) may well require one. You may want an advocate with you, someone to argue your case, or simply the comfort of a friend sitting close at hand; there will be no problem with this. Be ready to explain your situation as calmly as possible, and express your gratitude for the help they can give. If you can find the resources to be pleasant and appreciative, these qualities will go a long way towards your getting a sympathetic hearing. If you go in on a high horse demanding your rights, backs are likely to go up against you.

## Benefits

The social worker will help make sure that at all stages you and the brain damaged individual are getting all the help to which you are entitled. If you have power of attorney, the social worker should help you with completing the lengthy claim booklet for Disability Living Allowance (if under 65) or Attendance Allowance (if over 65) on your loved one's behalf. The care component of this cannot be paid while they are in hospital or residential care, but the mobility allowance is still payable, to offset costs of travelling to and from visiting. Payment of this can be backdated to the actual date when the disability came into play.

While it is usual nowadays for hospitals to make a considerable charge for visitor parking, there is often a system in place of reducing or even waiving these entirely in the case of a long stay. The average length of stay in hospital is something like three days; the charges certainly mount up when the stay turns into something like three months. Again the social worker – or even the charge nurse – should be able to help with information and arrangements around this. It may be down to you to ask in the first place, not because the authorities don't want you to have this help but simply because their minds are on other things and the need may well not have occurred to them.

Incapacity Benefit, Carer's Allowance and Child Tax Credit may also be available and your social worker will be up and running with current rules, rates and applicability. Nowadays, it is easy to make your own investigations via the Department for Work and Pensions website or helpline (see 'Useful addresses'). Remember that the Citizens' Advice Bureau is there for you too, in the case of any query or dispute.

Someone with 'severe mental impairment' is discounted as a resident for the purposes of council tax. Your GP will need to provide a certificate. She can also provide a certificate of exemption from prescription charges, which may save a large sum of money if a lot of medication is involved; for example, for the control of epilepsy.

There may be a range of smaller benefits available locally. For example, the local authority may offer discounted travel by public transport for those with a disability, which may also apply to a companion when one is necessary. They may also have a scheme for discounted access to leisure facilities in the locality. Your public library (as well as your social worker) is likely to be a useful source of information about these smaller but still valuable benefits.

## Cutting down on spending

At some time you are likely to need to take a long, hard look at your finances. It may be that cutting down on spending will be only the first part of the story; the second part being building up income. At some stage you may have to contemplate changing your job, or working longer hours, but that is for later. Try to focus on just one step at a time.

The household budget is always a balancing act – for some people easier to balance than for others. If your income is not meeting your expenditure, you have – broadly speaking – four options: to cut your expenditure, to increase your income, to do a bit of both, or to do nothing. The added difficulty now to this balancing act is the brain injury, which makes it impossible to look at your financial situation completely dispassionately. You will not yet know (indeed, no one can predict with certainty) how things will turn out, whether your loved one will manage to return to work, how far off such a return might be. If you are still in the thick of hospital visits, rehabilitation, perhaps occasional visits home with disability to adjust to, you are unlikely to have any energy – physical or emotional – to spare for boosting your income. It may be that the best you can do is decide not to worry about it for a certain period of time. Everything is dependent upon your own particular circumstances, but it is possible you may be able to enlist the help of a sympathetic bank manager if you can show that you are thinking sensibly about things.

For example, it is reasonable to assume that six months down the line you will have a clearer idea of your future circumstances. You are likely to have recovered to some extent from the shock of this sudden and extreme injury and things will be beginning to feel rather more stable. Provided you are the sort whose spending is not erratic, with a steady banking history behind you, a bank manager may well be minded to let you have an overdraft based on a reasonable estimate of your expenses. Or you may – because of exceptional circumstances and if you have a good record of meeting your payments – be granted a month or two's 'mortgage holiday'.This could give you the breathing space that you need; it may allow you to have a short break from work, while you give extra security to the children, make some input to your partner's rehabilitation and recover yourself. None of these things can be promised; but you can often get much further towards having what you want if you are prepared to ask nicely, discuss things openly and keep your nerve with the other parties involved.

But there may well be no way around it; at some point you are likely to have to cut your expenses. If you had an extravagant lifestyle before, your expenditure may reduce without you even trying. Expensive meals, weekends away and clothes shopping are likely to disappear off the agenda for a while. But other expenses may creep in – takeaways and convenience foods, treats for the children to lessen your bad feelings about having little time to spend with them at present, travel costs and parking charges for visiting the hospital.

If and when you do need to take steps to cut your expenditure, perhaps the best advice is, if you can, to do it in one fell swoop. There may come a point where you need to cut out a whole load of little pleasures. It's possible to save a lot by buying cheaper food, cutting out chocolate, alcohol, trips to the pub, the hiring of videos, the buying of CDs . . . But perhaps first it's worth considering doing something more drastic – perhaps laying up the car for six months so you have no insurance, road tax, AA membership, petrol or repairs to pay for. Or maybe you can do without the gym membership or the cleaner, the private healthcare or the dental plan. Memberships of pressure groups and political parties are worth looking at as a source of savings, as is insurance, which can be cut down to a bare minimum. After all, if you can cope when life has thrown *this* at you . . . !

In the end you may even need to economize on your children's activities, and if things must change for them they will adjust and get over their upset. But it may be worth trying to keep things as close to their normal routine as possible so as to give them some stability at a time when their security will have taken a severe rocking.

In all this working out about money, it is your attitude that will be the lifesaver. It may be that every financial adjustment has its bonus, its silver lining, but you will have to alter your mindset in order to see it. For example, there are benefits around not having a car, beyond the massive savings incurred. Greater fitness; freedom from sitting in traffic jams; the satisfaction of not contributing to pollution; escape from the fear that you might one day be responsible for a fatal accident. Certainly there are a lot of disadvantages to not having your own vehicle – but if you *need* to make that big saving, what is the point of focusing on them? Work to convince yourself instead of its benefits. It's to your advantage after all to stay positive if you can, rather than wallowing in misery.

Similarly, doing away with expensive holidays might mean you can take some time to explore the delights of countryside closer at hand. Doing without hotels can mean a lot of fun to be had camping, or in a youth hostel, meeting other people. These more primitive surroundings might be anathema to you – but if you're going to sulk over what you've lost, it's you who is going to be sunk in gloom. You may as well try to discover what other people find enjoyable in these things and other more homespun pleasures – it can do you no harm, and it may open up a whole new avenue in your life.

There is something of a trend nowadays, among a certain sector of society, towards *living better on less*. 'Downsizing' is all the rage. You too can follow the example of the burnt-out professionals in their forties who throw over their high-powered and highly paid jobs to live on a narrowboat or move to the country and grow their own vegetables. All right, so you may not yet have built your empire from which to downsize – but, if a lifestyle is desirable, why wait?

Nowadays the bulk of society seems to be made up of people who have either plenty of time or plenty of money. And it seems that the members of each group envy the members of the other! Perhaps we need to learn to appreciate what we've got – time or money – in whatever amount and make the most of it, rather than wasting our emotional energy in bouts of regret and envy. They are bound to arise, but we can actually help ourselves here with a bit of our own 'cognitive therapy'. When you catch yourself thinking along the lines of 'poor me' or 'lucky them', try bringing yourself to a definite stop. Make a positive effort then to call to mind all the things that you appreciate in your own life and dwell on these instead. With practice you will start to notice earlier in the process that you are heading towards the miserable land of 'if only' and eventually you may manage to train yourself to get to the point of stopping before you start. Contentment is a state of mind much sought after by practitioners of many different faiths – and for good reason; while it may smack of a cosy, stay-at-home, slippered mentality, it doesn't have to be anything of the sort.

Contentment is about finding pleasure and delight in the things that you have available to you in the present, instead of putting off your happiness until some future conditions have been met. We are very accustomed to being seduced by the advertising industry and television programmes into wanting all sorts of things that we do not actually need: holidays, fast cars, a stylish house, a beautifully laid-out garden. It becomes all too easy to imagine ourselves less fulfilled than others, even worse than others, if we don't have them and are not likely to be able to achieve them because of the circumstances of our lives.

But life is not a competition. We are entitled to live in the way we choose, the way that best fits with our personal circumstances, tastes and ethos – and we can do that, to a certain degree at least, whatever our income. All it takes is the self-belief that enables you to set yourself free from other people's standards, and the self-belief that allows you to set your own targets, define your own sources of pleasure and determine to relish the things of life that are available to you.

Perhaps this sounds very wishy-washy, perhaps it sounds very easy. In fact it is neither, particularly if you are not the naturally cheery, contented sort of person. But with determination and discipline you can go a long way in training yourself to enjoy to the full the things of the moment. What about that view, some time to sit and chat with friends, a burst of sunlight, or a good joke when there seems little around to laugh at? A baby's smile in a shop when you are feeling fraught about getting the shopping done, the pattern of frost on a windscreen, your loved one's physical presence and warmth however absent his mind? All too often we forget to enjoy the good things in life, because of our preoccupation with our problems and difficulties. Deciding to enjoy the good won't take the difficulties away. It won't make them any the less. But it will remind us that life is a rich mix of good and bad, delight and difficulty, and we do well to seize hold of everything to experience it fully. Let's determine not to give the negative the upper hand. The real joys of life are free for everyone to enjoy whatever their financial status. Once you start looking you may be surprised at their abundance.

# 8

## Psychological and emotional adjustments

None of us lives in isolation. We all belong to a range of communities: family, friends, work colleagues and residential neighbourhood. Just as the person who has suffered the brain injury is having to adjust to a different self, so each of these communities will be affected and changed to some extent. Other people will need to recognize and accept this new person too. If the injury is severe and the person who has suffered it has little insight into what has happened to them, it can be argued that the one most deeply affected by the injury is not the injured person but their nearest and dearest.

### *Realization and acceptance*

The nature of a brain injury is such that it can take an exceptionally long time for its dramatic impact on a person to be fully recognized and accepted by those who are very closely involved with them. If there is no visible evidence of an injury (if it was the result of internal damage, or the external wound has healed) it can be particularly difficult to accept the reality of the brain damage that has occurred.

Two things are arguing against this reality: your eyes, which are telling you that they *look* (more or less) all right and therefore must *be* all right; and your instinct for self-preservation, which is wanting to protect your own mind from having to acknowledge that such a terrible thing has happened. You may well experience a period of *denial* – though if you do you certainly won't recognize it as such until later. Others will need to be patient with you, and gentle in their discussions of what has happened and how your loved one is now, walking you little by little – following *your* pace – into its horrors and implications.

Denial can be an incredibly powerful mechanism. It can overcome enormously strong factual evidence of change. When in denial, it is perfectly possible, for example, to look at a wasted body in a wheelchair or someone in a coma with a drip, a catheter, and several monitors attached, and say with complete conviction, 'But there's nothing wrong with them!'

Denial can also be an elusive and contradictory mechanism, hard to pin down. Even in denial you may find it perfectly possible to discuss your loved one's acquired difficulties with a therapist, for example, and help carry out activities designed to improve the situation. There is no logic to it. It is simply your brain's way of coping with shock. Gradually, over time, denial has no choice but to melt away. Little by little you will have to acknowledge and face up to the difficulties that they now have.

'Realization', 'acknowledgement' and 'facing up to' are very different from acceptance. A refusal to accept what has happened can be a very useful source of energy in the battles that lie ahead. It can keep people going through very difficult times, and mean that the ultimate efforts are made towards someone's recovery at a time when those efforts are going to pay back the most. A stubborn and ongoing refusal to accept can fuel a determined continuation of the battle for improvement, long after others have been saying that no further recovery is possible.

But quite probably, acceptance or a refusal to accept are beyond the bounds of your own control. They will depend on your own emotional make-up, the quality of your relationship with the injured person, the circumstances of the injury, the other things going on in your life, and so on. As with realization, acceptance too will gradually come into play, whether you like it or not. Nobody can keep fighting for ever.

## Grieving – 'the living bereavement'

The person with a close friend or family member who has been seriously brain injured is suffering a bereavement. The person who was, is there no longer. And yet they are.

These are big and confusing issues to deal with. People meaning to be kind can unwittingly say the most upsetting things. 'Thank heavens she didn't die!' for example, when you are struggling with the notion that some things are worse than death. 'At least you've still got him', when the fact that you've got him means you've also got his memory problems, his fits, his incontinence, his irritability – though you've no longer got your shared past, his sense of humour, his sensitivity, his ability to calm your fears . . . and so on.

It is commonly agreed that the bereavement process takes about two years to go through. With a complicated bereavement such as this, the process is likely to take longer. You need time to grieve. But where are you going to find it when you are stuck in alongside the person whose departure you are grieving? How are you to grieve when you are caught up in such a mess of emotions that often you don't know whether to laugh (because they've survived) or cry (over what's happened to them)?

Time and space seem to be of the essence. Though it may go against the grain, perhaps you *should* take advantage of some offers of help and get away from the caring role for a while, however briefly. Give yourself permission to mourn what you have lost, to go over the past occasionally, celebrate what you had and grieve its passing. This does not have to be a self-pitying procedure. It is right to value what you had and important to acknowledge and mourn its loss. This process can also help to put the present reality and future possibilities into their true perspective.

Try if you can to find someone you can talk to honestly and openly about your feelings, someone whose shoulder you can cry on. Ideally, this would be a good friend, someone close to you, but they too may well be grieving, and if you are very confused it may be kinder and easier to seek some professional counselling help.

## Coping with loss – of friends

Unfortunately, the loss of your loved one as they used to be is generally not the only loss that brain injury brings with it. As if that wasn't bad enough, you may well lose others too. Some friends may disappear over time. Perhaps they find it too painful to see an old friend in their present state, or maybe they find it too difficult to cope with the effects of the brain injury. Or they and/or you may find it difficult to cope with the change in social circumstances that the brain injury demands.

For example, you may have been used to going round to another couple's for a meal occasionally, sharing long, intense conversations about current affairs or your favourite soap after the meal. But if an effect of the brain injury has been to make your partner insistent about telling and retelling the same few memories ad nauseam, refusing to allow anyone else to lead or contribute to a discussion, this sort of social occasion will simply become very trying for all involved.

Or perhaps you used to meet up with a group of friends for a rowdy night in the pub. If the brain injury has made hearing hypersensitive, or made it difficult to follow conversation in a group, the brain injured person may simply withdraw into themselves, or suffer a severe headache, or a bad temper outburst. No fun for anyone.

Sometimes social groups find it possible to adjust to include the brain damaged person. Sometimes they don't. Your friends might be willing to curtail the conversation and listen to music or play a board game instead. Or the invitations may become fewer and farther between. The group of friends you meet with may be willing to come round to your house instead with a few bottles, at least cutting out some of the background noise and giving a settled, familiar environment for the brain injured person.

But from your point of view, such adjustments may serve only to emphasize your loss. You might feel inclined to battle to hang on to things as they were, or you may consider it easier to take up an altogether different social activity. Over time you will have to accept that circumstances have now changed and it's very likely that your social life, perhaps even your circle of friends, will have to change with them.

## Loss of status

The brain injured person in many ways becomes very childlike, very dependent on others, without the wherewithal to rally arguments, to stick up for themselves, explore other possibilities in life, develop new talents, or even quite likely explain their behaviour (which can be embarrassing or challenging) or difficulties (which can be hard for others to grasp). And to add insult to injury, it's quite likely that the person who has suffered the injury doesn't seem to care; they may be lost in a sort of limbo-land without any drive or motivation to get out.

Brain injury is no respecter of status. The individual's former position – perhaps long held – in professional circles, socially, or even just within the family is suddenly whisked away. Respect can quickly be replaced by embarrassment, awkwardness, shame or laughter – however many kind attempts are made to pretend otherwise. Depending on your relationship with the injured person there may well be a knock-on effect for you. Even if it is only their loss of status that you feel, it may well be felt severely, and all the more so because they are unaware of it themselves.

The loss of status is also a loss of potential. Along with the person who was and their achievements, have gone the person who was to be and their future. Your hopes and dreams for the future will all have to be reassessed. But don't be hard on yourself – they don't need to be reassessed today. You may both have more of a future ahead of you than it would seem at this point.

Once again you will need to bring into play the ability to live one day at a time, allowing space to come to terms with what has happened and for the pain to ease.

## *Loss of a sex life*

If it is your partner who has suffered the brain injury, you may find – and you may be surprised to find – that the loss of your sex life is one of the hardest things you have to deal with. It is not of course a loss you will feel immediately. But as the period of severe anxiety recedes and things begin to settle into a slower pace, you may well begin to feel it very strongly.

Some people feel sexual frustration as a fierce pain, some as a dull ache. And for many people, depending on their age, their social groupings and taboos, it is a pain that they feel obliged to suffer in silence.

We all have an inbuilt appetite for sex, and once we have become accustomed to having this appetite regularly satisfied in a stable adult relationship, our bodies will cry out in hunger until they readjust to going without. Masturbation can help ease the pain during this time of readjustment and is only natural.

Over time, though, as the pain lessens, a practice which has previously offered some comfort often begins only to emphasize the loss. Whereas the physical appetite is becoming less urgent, the emotional appetite for physical intimacy with another human being remains just as strong, and is an appetite that masturbation cannot satisfy. At this stage you may begin to find that indulging in this practice leaves you feeling only deeply upset. It's time then to try if you can to leave it behind; perhaps you can manage to distract yourself with other activities when you feel tempted.

You may be surprised to receive unsolicited advice from friends or others, suggesting you should look around for sexual satisfaction from someone else. You may even receive an approach from someone who, knowing your situation, may feel they are offering some much needed help. You may feel deeply insulted by this advice or by such an approach. Or you may be tempted to take that route. You may just happen, around this time, to meet someone to whom you feel a strong physical attraction, and who might well reciprocate. Perhaps another sexual relationship beckons.

Assuming the possible relationship would be with someone otherwise unattached, the only person with any right to blame you for following this route would be yourself. For precisely this reason, tread very carefully. You already have a heavy emotional load to carry. Be careful that you know your own mind. Be clear about your motives, about any possible entanglements that might follow, and about your ability to deal with what is very likely to be a further emotional complication. If you do start down this road, be ready to take steps towards backing out the minute anything starts to feel amiss. Few people – particularly women, it has to be said – manage to separate sex and emotion entirely successfully. If you are serious about retaining an emotional involvement with your loved one, however badly brain damaged, it may in the long run be easier if you can to accept the celibate life.

## Other losses

A variety of losses is associated with brain injury, as with any acquired disability. You need to take these losses seriously. Make sure you acknowledge how much they hurt, and grieve them. As with everything else, this will be a process. It does not involve wallowing in self-pity. It does involve expressing your sorrow, whether to friends, family, stranger-professionals, or in tears on your pillow at dead of night.

Eventually, if you are not to become bitter and twisted, you will need to come to terms with your losses. One exercise that may help involves starting from a position of believing that you have lost everything. Try to convince yourself that you have nothing in life. No friends, no status, no income (worth having), no choice, no opportunity, no hope. I trust you will find this difficult! From this perspective, thoughts should come flooding in to remind you just what a wealth of valuable assets you do have. For example, these may include loving family members, (some) supportive friends, (sufficient) money to live comfortably, opportunities to work, to learn, the chance to follow leisure pursuits, a pleasant home. You may not have as much of any of these as you had before, your circumstances may indeed be reduced, your losses may be significant – but looking at life from the perspective of a glass half-full rather than the glass half-empty is always going to feel better.

## Coping with routine

Obviously this brain injury is going to have an impact on your routine, and that sounds like an easy adjustment to make. We all have to make changes to our routines at various stages of life: when we change our jobs, when we take on a pet or an evening class, when we go on holiday, and so on. We can appreciate the point of the routine – we need to do A now in order to have time to do B later; or we need to feed the dog now in order that he's not chewing the house to pieces later, and so on. There's a logic to it that we can see – though the very fact of things being routine means that we don't need to consider the logic every time we do routine tasks (which would slow us down); we can just get on and do them and that's that.

But routine is different for people with memories that don't work very well. Have you ever found yourself wondering whether you've cleaned your teeth or fed the dog already? Routine tasks can be done on automatic while our minds are elsewhere. And routine can be – and is for us too – an aid to memory. If we wonder whether we've cleaned our teeth, the chances are that we have, because we are so used to going automatically from one task to the other that we scarcely notice. The same is true for the person with a brain injury. Though they may not have laid down a memory in their mind, or may not be able to call it up, it's as if the body itself has some level of memory of its own. By being trained to follow the same sequence of actions over and over it becomes automatic, and so long as someone prompts the beginning of the sequence, the brain injured person may more or less reliably be expected to follow it through to the end. If you play a musical instrument, you may appreciate this notion easily. When you learn a piece of music 'by heart', it's as if your fingers know which way they are expected to go without having to refer to the memory itself between the playing of each note.

So routine has a particular place in the life of the brain injured person. It can help them to carry out necessary tasks with more ease, such as getting up in the morning, using the sequence of washing, cleaning teeth, putting on clothes and shoes and going downstairs. As with anything where brain injury is concerned, building up the routine in the first place can be a very long and slow process, but over time it is likely to be a considerable aid to independence in some part of the day at least.

'Structure', or a shape to the day, is also helpful. It's an unusual person who lives an unstructured life. Each day is broken into morning, afternoon and evening, which for almost everyone are structured by mealtimes and working shifts. Events or activities within each part of the day may vary, but there will be a certain element of predictability. Although we may not do the same thing every morning, mornings have a similar shape, in that we get up at their beginning and have a certain range of tasks to carry out before the morning ends with lunch.

For all of us routine and structure are helpful. They enable us to do boring things with less effort, and they enable us to move from task to task without undue mental input and physical/mental upset. But whereas most of us have the flexibility to break away from routine and structure where this is either necessary or desirable, for the brain injured person this is extremely difficult.

The brain injured person is likely to want to get up at the same time every day, will take exactly the same amount of time to go through their morning routine, unable to adjust to any particular element of rush or relaxation that this particular day requires or allows. If an appointment beckons it will be hard to leave the house earlier than usual; if it's been a particularly busy week for the household, it will be difficult to take it more slowly come Saturday morning. Whereas you might be accustomed to skip lunch on a busy day, even a delay to the usual mealtime might be hard for a brain injured person to accept.

Practically speaking this need for routine is likely to be something you will have to take on board. Depending to some extent on the temperament of the brain injured individual, it may be that the life of the whole household will need to revolve around this one person's need for a very rigid routine. There will always be occasions when routine simply has to go to pot, but it may be worth the effort to keep such occasions to a minimum in order to avoid emotional upset and the consequences of that for other family members. Even if the brain injured person is not severely angered or frustrated by upsets to routine, there will always be an element of tension between your desire sometimes to throw routine out of the window and their need to retain it at virtually all costs. Probably only you can discover how to cope with this tension and how far you will need to adjust your own way of life in order to accommodate this effect of the brain injury.

## Life's rhythms

Before the brain injury you might well have measured the rhythms of your life in terms of time spent out at work and time spent at home – your 'own time'. Suddenly you have responsibility of a different order for this other person. Your own routine and rhythm of life are going to be different now whether or not you have adopted the role of full-time carer. Even if you continue to go out to work there is going to be an element of care – even if only 'supervision' – in your life. There is much more call now upon your 'own time' and the feelings around being out at work and being at home may become blurred. You may find that going out to work feels like the release that coming home felt like before, and that work is therapeutic in a way that it was not previously. Leisure may be a commodity in very short supply.

You may well have to adjust too to the fact that care workers come into your home. This may not bother you. If you are the gregarious sort, you may positively welcome their presence, particularly if you find the individuals concerned likeable. If on the other hand you like to be private, having to let 'strangers' in to work in your own living accommodation, giving them access to your own belongings and care over your own loved one may be very difficult for you to accept.

In practical terms you probably have little choice. You may well need to continue working either for financial reasons or for emotional ones (whether a psychological need to work, or a need to get away from this brain injury for a large part of each day – which may amount to the same thing). If so, you are unlikely to have any other option but to use home care to some extent. If this tension is there for you, all you can probably do to help is acknowledge that you dislike these arrangements and perhaps offload some of your annoyance onto a sympathetic ear. But if this tension is the downside of a more amenable overall picture then you will need – and want – to come to terms with it. Over time you will of course become used to the idea; it will cease to concern you, and will become part of the (abnormal) normality of your daily life.

It may happen that on occasion you need to be at home while care workers are there too. You may find it difficult to relax when your home is someone else's workspace, or when your home hours are filled with all the business of managing a brain injury, running a household, organizing family matters and all the associated financial, educational and health arrangements. If you can, set up a place in your home as your own private space. It might be a spare room or simply a corner of your bedroom or dining room. Try to make it an area that the care workers do not need to use, and put in a little effort to set it up in a way that supports or at least reflects your need for – and right to – your own private life. Even if only in very small ways, make it amenable to your own distinctive tastes. It might be a place you need to use to manage the household affairs, where you sit down to pay the bills, and so on. But you can still put a favourite picture on the wall, maybe have a CD or cassette player with some of *your* music to hand. Make a little effort to comfort yourself – it's surprising just how the slightest things can go towards making life bearable.

If arrangements can be made for regular periods of respite care, this may form the basis of a new rhythm to your life. To begin with, you may find respite difficult to handle. There can be quite a tangle of emotions around it. You will probably have been looking forward to this first break, saving things up to do while the brain injured person is away. Perhaps you have even, on occasion, been wishing your loved one out of the way. Then when it comes to it, you may find you can hardly bear to let them go, worried about how they will cope in a strange setting and without you. Or you might feel guilty about wishing them gone and relishing your own free time. And in the event, you may find it difficult to adjust to the brain injured person's absence, hard to put your mind to the things you were so looking forward to doing, distracted by anxieties about your loved one, or suddenly overwhelmed with emotions you had been holding at bay in their presence.

All these are entirely natural feelings and only to be expected. But no one is likely to speak about these sorts of difficulties. And it is hard to explain even to well-meaning and sympathetic family and friends what a welter of emotions is associated with the partings and meetings of someone you love with a disability you hate for coming between you. So in the end you learn to say nothing, opting (though not really by choice) to stay in isolation, since no one really understands.

Accepting this sense of isolation can be dangerous. You need to find some sort of outlet for your emotions if at all possible. If you have nowhere safe to express them, a process of displacement might be better than nothing. People channel negative emotions into all sorts of things. Some people vent anger or frustration in hard physical exertion, running or going to the gym. Some people find help in more meditative activities such as yoga or going for long walks. Others are able to channel their feelings into art, or express them, however directly or otherwise, in poetry, story or music.

## Building a new relationship

After several months or more of having the professionals looking in on you, there's a danger that this relationship itself might become institutionalized! If you are serious about staying in it, you will want to make it work, on whatever level. It won't be able to work as it worked before. Before, it will have operated in many different modes, to suit different periods of life, different aspects of your days together – physical, emotional, practical, work, leisure, light-hearted, serious, and so on. Now, it is likely that the extent and range of that relationship is vastly reduced, so that you can operate together only in much more limited ways.

Your relationship is likely to be much more limited. It may well also be very changed. After all, this is in many ways a new person to whom you are now relating. And there is a tension too between being someone's carer – particularly when their behaviour, their thought processes and their conversation are unorthodox – and having a properly personal relationship with them.

On the one hand you will need to accept these changes and limitations or be seriously frustrated. On the other, if the relationship is to survive, you will probably need to push the boundaries in order to set it once again on a more personal level. After months of illness and rehabilitation, it may even take a while before you can feel properly relaxed in their presence at home. You will probably need to make a positive effort to have a private life together, taking the initiative in embarking on any intimate behaviour, whether this is physical, or in the form of sharing private memories from your past lives together, looking over old photos for example, expressing your love for the person who has now gone. This process in itself may help you discover more points of connection with the person they now are. This relationship has suffered a severe setback and is being re-established on new terms. Even if all the growth and development have to take place on your side, it will still be sufficient for its survival.

# 9
## Your life together

Life with a newly brain injured person can be very unpredictable. It may feel quite scary at the beginning as you assume a higher level of responsibility for this person's well-being. You may have big ideas about what you are going to achieve, the route you are going to follow and the destination you intend to reach. But – unless you have an unusual amount of foresight – the journey will probably not go as you plan.

As this new life becomes familiar, as things settle down and a routine becomes established, your future together may begin to loom rather large in your mind. Before the injury, whatever time you were accustomed to spending together was probably busy and satisfying. You would have been making plans, spoken or unspoken, and had your individual and shared challenges, interests and desires. You would have been growing alongside each other, and growing your relationship between you. Suddenly, it is all down to you. Perhaps the future now seems to pan out before you as an alarming conglomeration of unfilled and unfulfilled days, weeks, months, years.

You still want – and need – to grow. But your loved one? It's likely that they seem to have come to a standstill.

That's probably an illusion. Doctors may put a time limit on the recovery from a brain injury, warning you to expect no more progress after a certain period of time. Yet there are many people, family members and experts among them, who consider that the brain continues to heal itself for the rest of its life. The trouble is, though, that this healing and the resulting personal development progress at such a slow rate that it usually feels as if there is no movement at all. The early recovery, which even then seemed fearsomely slow, will seem like lightning by comparison. We are now looking at the slightest of changes that take place over many months, if not years – changes that often become apparent only when we look back to how things once were.

You will need to keep yourself going through these months and years, trying to maintain an overview of the situation so that you don't become completely disheartened. You will also need to find motivation enough to keep *the two of you* going at any efforts you are making to retrain, re-engage and rehabilitate. It is unlikely that your loved one can recall yesterday's challenge successfully achieved. They can't plan how to build on that success, or work out where they want to be in two years' time and define the various steps on the way. And it's unlikely they can weigh up the pros and cons of making a further effort versus sitting back and doing nothing.

The most vital resource for supplying this motivation will be the conviction that what you are doing is worthwhile. And if you are going to be able to maintain this motivation and support for such long periods of time, it will need to feel worthwhile not only for the brain injured person but for you too. If you are not to become bitter, you will need to have your own reason for this relationship to survive, in whatever form.

This may sound harsh. It may sound ridiculous to you. 'She's my mother, for goodness' sake!' I hear you cry. Or 'He's my husband! I'm not going to walk away from him.' No one here is suggesting that you should. The suggestion is rather that it is worth examining your reasons for continuing to support this person, whether you are giving up your own career to become a full-time carer, or planning to continue visiting them in their care home twice-weekly on an ongoing basis.

If you are able to look at the whole situation as objectively as possible, considering the extent of the brain injury and the impact it is having on both your lives (and the lives of other family members); if you can understand your own needs in this situation and the needs of your loved one, and work out how best these can all be dovetailed together . . . then for the time being at least you should have found a workable solution.

There will be people who seek to help by foisting their own solutions onto you, what they would or wouldn't do if they found themselves in a similar situation. But the fact is that this is you, not them. If you know that you would be driven out of your mind with boredom if you adopted the role of full-time carer, then nobody should make you feel guilty (intentionally or unintentionally) about a decision to maintain your own career and use residential or home care for the injured person. It would not be a healthy situation for anybody if you were to stay home harbouring resentment or repressing anger at feeling trapped in a situation that doesn't suit your temperament. Over time, things would eventually come to the boil and some sort of crisis arise, probably to the permanent damage of the relationship. Similarly, if you know that you could not live with yourself if you were to walk out on this relationship, whatever it is (and there are very likely to be people around advising you to do just that), then that is important too. And there is of course a whole range of diverse options between these two extremes.

Try to spend some time in a serious attempt to make honest, real and hard decisions about how you want to live your life, rather than letting yourself drift into a situation. Make space to work out not how other people want you to live in these new circumstances, but how you want to live in them. Over time, this process will save you a lot of emotional energy. Knowing where you stand and what you really want to do will help you not to become emotionally confused and distracted when other people present you with their own ideas. And probably more importantly, when the going gets tough – and it most surely will – you can refer back to the reasons why you are living in the way you are. You will be able to remind yourself of the basis of your decisions, acknowledge the difficulties you are going through and give yourself credit for continuing despite them for the greater good that you have in sight.

No decision though is made for ever, and this too is important to remember. Remind yourself that this is the way you have decided to operate *for now*. It might be beneficial too to decide to review that decision once a year, say. This can help tide you through sticky patches. It can ensure that you don't just chuck in the towel because, for example, you have temporarily come under the negative influence of a new acquaintance or you are going through a period of frustration which could be relieved by some respite. We all have 'higher selves' and, though for much of the time our emotions and moods may hold more sway over the way we behave, going against our best instincts does not in the end lead to happiness or fulfilment.

So having made the decision – for now – to stay with this relationship, how are you going to cope? There are certain things you can do that will not only benefit your loved one's continuing rehabilitation, but will also make things more bearable and satisfying for you – even if, in the first instance, they may not be easy to set up. Yes, you may well need the motivation of two people – that is, if the brain injured person has no motivation of their own, you may need to motivate yourself and them too in order to get the two of you out and doing. But it will be worth it.

## Bringing interest into your lives

You have gone through a period of time in which there has, frankly, been altogether too much interest in your life. For some time you are likely to have been riding the emotional roller coaster of serious and incapacitating illness and working the treadmill of hospital visiting, appointments with specialists and therapists on top of all your other responsibilities.

When the time finally comes when all this stops it may feel as though it has all stopped quite suddenly. Almost as if you have been through a storm, a shipwreck, and here you are marooned on a desert island with someone who is – there is no denying it – 'rather strange'. Someone who is unable to give you the emotional comfort that you need, to pick up the clues of how you are feeling and respond helpfully. Someone who may need more or less constant supervision in order to keep them safe, who may get exceedingly angry – even violent – when frustrated, who perhaps repeats themselves endlessly throughout the day, or demands your attention every minute. You are likely to feel isolated. However many people are around you, you are on your own in this situation in which your personal relationship with this individual has been so very damaged. No one else can fully know just what you have lost, nor can they properly appreciate the difficulties you are struggling with in this new relationship. Many of these are hard to measure objectively and may depend on things that vary, such as mood, situation, the reaction and behaviour of other people. Some of the difficulties you are experiencing may depend on the working together of your two specific personalities. From outside the relationship many of the problems may be invisible, certainly to those beyond the immediate family and the professionals who can ask the right questions.

There comes a point where you are going to have to address this sense of isolation for the sake of your own sanity. A few hours of respite care a week, or whatever it is that you get, is all well and good and not to be done without, but on top of that you need to try to put the rest of the week's hours into a better perspective. Seek to confront this sense of isolation, or sense of purposelessness, or boredom – whatever the emotion is that is getting you down – and try to do something about it. In other words, bring something into your life together that can be of benefit to you both.

## So what can you do? Setting goals

Instead of drifting along from day to day as if on a permanent holiday, working to some sort of agenda can put your whole life into a better perspective. Even the achievement of small targets can provide satisfaction and overcome hopelessness by marking progress.

For example, you may decide that it would be worth both your whiles to become more physically fit. You will need to decide on the ultimate goal, which may be a five-mile walk, swimming ten lengths or taking part in a wheelchair sports event. The targets on the way to achieving the goal might be quite varied. They may include such things as saving up for a particular piece of equipment or clothing, finding out where and how you can join a particular sporting group, setting out a progressive training schedule, and so on. Each target gives you something to look forward to, to work towards, some sense of satisfaction on its achievement and a reason for putting certain activities – preferably something that you both enjoy doing – into each day.

The hardest part will be for you to remain determined and motivated for the two of you through the whole process. When your other half doesn't ever want to make the effort for themselves, there's no one else around to say to you, 'Oh come on, let's keep trying.' You have to do that bit for yourself, and even at times when your resources are very low. And the pay-off for all the effort can seem exceedingly small, especially if you have to celebrate alone.

Nor is it always easy to work out what the goals could be. The starting point may as well be your own emotions. Consider what emotion you are really struggling with. If it's boredom and lack of energy, physical exercise can turn things around wonderfully. If it's frustration or upset, consider what is most upsetting or frustrating about your new circumstances. It's likely to be something that feels enormous – enormous and unchangeable. And in its entirety it might be. But perhaps by breaking the enormous thing down into its constituent parts, you might find you can work to improve one small part and make it feel that little bit less terrible.

The frustration may be as enormous as the fact that they are *always there*. Over time you might just be able to win yourself a small break in the day by teaching your wife how to go to the corner shop (or the postbox, or a friend's house) safely on her own. You need to break this goal down into small steps and expect to take a long time to achieve each one.

The first step might be to walk with her to the corner shop every day for two weeks. Identify some landmarks on the way, and point these out to her each day in the same sequence and in the same way, lodging them into her memory. Assuming she can read, write down the route to the shop, including the landmarks that you have familiarized her with. If not she will need to learn the landmarks off by heart, ticking them off mentally as she passes them. Continue to walk with her to the shop, but now making sure she has the directions in her hand. Keep reminding her to refer to them. Then move towards walking some way behind her to the shop, watching how she follows the directions and seeing if she can do this safely on her own.

Eventually the time comes when you need to risk letting her step out on her own. Although she seems to have the knowledge securely with you, you will notice the time she leaves and be on edge until her safe return – and if she doesn't return at the expected time, off you go quickly to find out where she has got to. If she hasn't quite managed it this time, go back a step or two and persevere again.

An exercise such as this can have beneficial results for you both; your wife will have an increased sense of independence and self-respect, and you will have earned a short breather in the days now when she goes to the shop by herself. A small achievement perhaps – but with many possibilities to be built on.

It may be that you find you get irritated with your loved one's difficulties, and then feel bad about yourself. Perhaps every day your husband gets himself dressed but always needs reminding to put on his shoes before going out. Perhaps he goes regularly to a day centre, and always at the last minute you realize that he still has his slippers on; the transport is waiting outside, you get irritated, he gets upset, the transport is kept waiting and the day always starts off on the wrong foot. Your goal will be to get him to the point where he remembers to put his shoes on himself.

You might start by leaving a note, 'Please put your shoes on', in the first place he goes to when he gets downstairs. Assuming he is biddable, he will turn round, go back upstairs and put his shoes on. After a couple of weeks of this, you might start prompting him before he goes downstairs with the question, 'What are you going to find when you get downstairs?' At first you may need to supply the answer, but eventually he will know the answer himself, and finally will think of the question and answer himself and begin to put his shoes on instead of his slippers without any prompting at all. One small step towards reducing your irritation levels and making for an easier start to the day. It has taken a lot of effort, but is probably worth it.

It is impossible to give examples of helpful goals and their associated targets to fit every single set of circumstances, when they are so wide-ranging. You will need to look creatively at your own lives, refusing to be defeated. Encourage yourself by focusing always on the progress that has been made, however small, rather than on the enormity of the distance still to cover. Remember, as Desmond Tutu pointed out, that the way to eat an elephant is one mouthful at a time!

## Finding activities

If money is in short supply the opportunities for activities to provide more interest, challenge, light and shade in your lives may seem very limited. They may indeed be harder to find, and they may be more difficult to engage in when one of you has a brain injury. But with determination, they are there to be found.

Many community groups will welcome you and your disability as volunteers. There are environments where people are willing – even required – to be accommodating and inclusive for the benefit of all. Though you may feel disabled as a couple, with your shared difficulties and abilities adding up sometimes to less than even one fully able person, you can still be a bonus to a group. With you there alongside the brain injury, with your knowledge of how best to manage it, many things become possible, always depending of course on the temperament and outlook of the injured person and the willingness of an organization to be flexible to your needs.

One of those needs is likely to be the chance to engage very gradually with the new activity, group and environment. You may only be able to stay for ten minutes on the first visit. It may take six months or more before you can really begin to enjoy or benefit from it. You may have to be persuasive, even assertive, in the first instance, to convince those in positions of power that what you want to achieve is a good idea and that they should open the door for you to carry it out. Increased numbers of people living with brain injury are a fact of modern society, and it is as well for any organization worth its salt to take this on board.

If people can be persuaded to be sympathetic, here are just a few of the opportunities that you could investigate:

- help in a charity shop;
- serve teas, lunches in a day centre – or help to clear up after the session;
- stuff envelopes etc. for political parties/pressure groups/charitable organizations;
- write pro forma letters for Amnesty International;
- go litter picking/tree-planting/collecting goods for recycling with an environmental group;
- deliver a community newsletter or advertising fliers.

Activities such as these can benefit you (as well as the organization you are helping) in two ways. First of all, it's good for your self-esteem to be making a contribution. On top of that, just having been out somewhere and in contact with someone – however little you may have felt inclined to do those things at the time – can serve to put your hours at home into a completely different and much more attractive perspective.

Nowadays far more leisure opportunities are open to disabled people, many offered by local councils at a discount. However, you may well find that the nature of the particular disabilities you are involved with are a bar to many of these. Memory problems rob the cinema and theatre, for example, of most of their appeal. But sport can be enjoyable – for both of you – and so can music. If opportunities are limited, you may need to determine to enjoy even the slightest of pleasures. Working your way systematically through the cassettes on loan at your local library, for example, is hardly exciting stuff. But it provides a reason to leave the house, gives you a little fresh air and exercise and the chance of some social contact. And while back at home your beloved may simply enjoy the music in the moment, you can be turning yourself into an expert on the differences between salsa and reggae, folk songs from various parts of the world, or the classics.

Some local councils operate special sessions at the pool for disabled people, sometimes for free, or at a reduced rate. These may or may not feel appropriate in your circumstances. If your situation does not involve any great or obvious physical disability, you may feel uncomfortable taking your place among those who need hoists to get in and out of the water, or embarrassed at swimming lengths when others may only be able to float. On the other hand, if the brain injury means that crowds are difficult to cope with, a lot of noise is upsetting, or collisions in a busy pool are difficult to avoid, using the pool when it is quieter is perfectly justifiable. You too may find it less stressful to embark on this activity in the company of people who are accustomed to challenging behaviour, to outbursts of anger or loud hilarity – people who are accustomed to taking others entirely as they find them.

The local gym can also be a place of recreation. It may not have appealed to you before. But with this less active lifestyle that has more or less been forced on you, perhaps the time has come to be ready to take what you can get. At a discount, and without the highly competitive pressure that some people insist on putting on them-selves, half an hour or so at the gym two or three times a week could prove to be a pleasant and sociable interlude, with the bonus of increased fitness. Physical exercise is also a very good way of making the brain more alert, and is certainly helpful in maintaining general mental health, for both of you.

It can be hard to maintain the positive attitude necessary to get involved in these sorts of activities. In the first place, you may make all this effort for your loved one's benefit. But some of these activities can have spin-offs for you too. At the swimming group, for example, there is the chance for you to meet with others who will understand your predicament, with others who are also likely to want some social contact. In voluntary work, it may be that, as your loved one becomes familiar with the setting and routines and as others become used to their ways, someone else will keep an eye on them for a short time and give you the occasional break. Or you too may develop new skills, find pleasure in this sort of outlet, and become aware of other opportunities and choices in life.

## Staying on top

A wealth of advice on how to cope with the various difficulties resulting from a brain injury is available from the various brain injury associations (see 'Useful addresses'). But be sure too to trust your own instincts. Keep an open mind when listening to advice, being ready to weigh its merits, and to try it out if it seems worthwhile. But always remember that brain injury is individual – you know this person and their brain injury better than anyone else and this counts for a lot.

Remember too that the introduction of any new management system is likely to need some time before it can become established. For example, teaching someone with memory problems to use a diary can take a matter of months, or longer, and even then may never become really secure. Unless you have someone else's involvement and encouragement it can be hard to engage in programmes of retraining that demand a huge amount of emotional energy from you. Words of advice on paper have their place, but if you are really struggling with particular difficulties the best port of call might be the GP, to see whether he can offer a referral for some more back-up.

Sometimes the most helpful way of tackling the difficulty is not concerned with changing the behaviour of the brain injured individual, but with changing your attitude to that behaviour. Sometimes you may need to acknowledge that there is a particular battle that you're not going to win, and for the sake of your own sanity or blood pressure you need to turn away from it. It may be, for example, that at every slightest mention of religion, your wife launches into an account of her conversion experience, however inappropriate. You may have tried all sorts of methods to change this behaviour: persuasion, diversion, distraction, prevention, deterrence (with anger perhaps), but nothing has had any effect.

Meanwhile your emotional temperature continues to rise with every failed attempt to prevent this happening. It can't get much higher without something giving. Perhaps it would be best to switch your efforts from trying unsuccessfully to change your wife's behaviour into trying to change your own response to it. After all, it is you who is suffering the most in this situation; your wife clearly doesn't mind, and anyone else she is relating the story to can afford to be indulgent. Yes, they may think her a little strange, they may be a bit mystified – they may even be interested! Two things are certain: the story won't have the strength of impact for them that it has for you, and they won't have to hear the story anything like the number of times you do.

So, make up your mind that at the first sign of her starting on that line of conversation you will focus your mind on . . . on what? It can be anything at all, but preferably something tranquil. Perhaps you might relive a particularly happy occasion or go through a mental catalogue of wild birds you have spotted locally. Perhaps you could focus on some project you have ongoing, the plot of a story you are writing or the redecoration of the bathroom, or you could try recalling the twists and turns of a film you enjoyed recently. You can use anything that will be an attractive distraction for you. And if at first you don't succeed, keep trying; your concentration will improve with practice.

Bringing this sort of strategy into play is not an admission of defeat. It's more like engaging the SAS in an act of subterfuge. A large part of what you are fighting for is the survival of your relationship. If you can switch off emotionally from whatever particular type of behaviour is really bugging you it's got to be better for the overall picture. Once you have switched off emotionally from it, you may also then find yourself better able to think it through in a logical way and come up with fresh ideas as to how to tackle it.

Another useful strategy in your ongoing life together may be the enlistment of alternative therapies. An increasing number of people seem to find one or more of them helpful in dealing with the stresses and strains of daily life. Such things as massage, aromatherapy and reflexology may prove helpful, largely as an aid to relaxation, for either one or both of you.

Be cautious though about the claims made regarding the benefits of some of the more unusual treatments, and don't go into any of these things with high hopes for further healing. That way you won't be disappointed. It would be wise in any case to check with the GP or specialist for their opinion of any particular therapy before starting a course, as well as checking the credentials of the practitioner. For yourself, many local authorities now offer specially arranged days for carers, often including taster sessions in a range of alternative therapies.

# 10

# Your own life

## *Moving on*

The reason you are prepared to invest so much time, effort and emotional energy in this person's recovery and rehabilitation is probably that your lives have been bound together for a long time. At some point, though, you are going to recognize the need to move on in your own life, to separate yourself to some extent emotionally from the brain injured person, opening yourself up to new experiences that will not be shared.

From your present standpoint, you may view this notion with horror. But unless you can eventually make such a move, your relationship is likely to be doomed. It would simply not be possible for anyone to sustain a relationship indefinitely with a severely brain injured person without finding from somewhere the fulfilment – intellectual, spiritual, emotional – that feeds and nurtures them as an individual. You will still need to grow, to experience life, to learn – and the harsh fact is that whereas before you probably did much of this together, now you will need to do it for yourself.

If you decide this is what you will do, to embark on adult education courses, learn a musical instrument, go to the theatre or concerts, seek out congenial company, go on long walks – whatever it is that sustains you – then you will be in control of the situation. You will return to your caring role refreshed, invigorated, with things to think and talk about and feeling fulfilled as a person. If you don't make this sort of move, but try to ignore the tension and tie yourself down to the level and limitations of the brain injury, you will over time become very vulnerable to having your life hijacked. You might easily fall prey to mental illness, to a religious cult, to an unwanted sexual approach, and have your life and emotions spiral away out of your control. Even if none of these things happen, you will eventually be leading a dull and dreary life, unsatisfying for you and unhelpful for the brain injured person too; a recipe for disaster on all fronts.

## *Claiming your own life*

What with taking up voluntary work and sporting activities, meeting up with friends, working out goals and targets, structuring the day to build a routine that will accommodate all those necessary daily tasks and making the most of other local opportunities, you're going to be kept pretty busy. Finding the motivation and energy to keep two people going, particularly when the other person cannot manage to throw routine out of the window for a day off, and particularly when all the effort is being focused on someone else's long-term benefit, can be hard. It might begin to feel like one long obstacle course, a treadmill on which you must keep working with an enforced smile and positive attitude.

At some point you will need to make what might seem like a subtle shift in attitude. It simply involves reminding yourself, 'This is my life as well.'

Inside the home you may get along pretty well. Over time you are likely to have found some activities that your loved one can engage in with a minimal level of supervision or support, such as watching television or videos, playing computer games, doing puzzle books. Meanwhile you can do your own thing, connected to the outside world occasionally by the radio or the phone and switched off to some extent from their problems.

But you can't be at home all the time. When you are out together, everything may be experienced differently. You may suddenly catch yourself seeing through the eyes of the onlooker, the one who is trying to puzzle out the situation unfolding before their eyes. You become the ticket inspector watching you treat a grown man like one of your children. Or the shop assistant startled by a very loud and dirty laugh over something totally innocuous in which there is apparently a deeply hidden innuendo. You feel the mortification of the whole group when your husband suddenly makes to display his private parts. The embarrassment can be acutely painful.

Perhaps you have the opportunity to go on an outing to a place you have wanted to visit for a long time, or a place that means a lot to you. You are really looking forward to this, to soaking up the atmosphere of the place, to some relaxation, or to taking your time to explore and get to know somewhere special. But when it comes to it your loved one is uncooperative, unable to appreciate anything of the visit, disorientated by the strange surroundings and uneasy at being in a different place, put on edge by the noise, desperate for the loo, or wanting unending cups of coffee. Whatever it is, the trip has not gone as you were hoping. It's not been the treat you were looking forward to. The difficulties have ruined the day, made it not worth the effort, and you have come home more frazzled than ever.

Perhaps one glorious day you decide to go for a country walk. But his endlessly repetitive chatter or incessant questioning about where you are and what you are going to do afterwards rob the event of any pleasure. You come back wound up like a coiled spring.

You will come to expect the pain and tension of embarrassment, irritation and frustrated pleasure and look for some way of coping with them. Some people use avoidance as a strategy. They keep away from company, stop planning outings they would otherwise enjoy, or plan to engage in certain activities only on their own, while the brain injured person is in respite care or staying with friends or family.

But avoidance is not very satisfactory. It makes your own life so much smaller, limits the pleasure that you are able to receive by engaging in new experiences, restricts the variety of your days and cuts down your social contact. If you're not careful, avoidance can become a way of life, bringing some nasty characters along in its wake – anxiety, agoraphobia, depression.

Much better to work out strategies that will enable you to keep living life to the full, albeit with some amount of compromise. Try to make a realistic assessment of the level at which the two of you are able to engage in certain social situations. For example:

- a meal in a restaurant or café;
- doing the shopping;
- time on the beach;
- an evening in the pub with friends.

It might be, for example, that whereas *you* could enjoy some time relaxing on the beach, your loved one could not cope with the aimless hours, the absence of a proper chair, or the crowds of people. Rather than denying yourself the beach altogether, how would it be if you travelled a bit further to a quieter place, invested in a decent folding chair and took a puzzle book along?

Doing the shopping might be a weekly ordeal for you. But rather than setting it aside to cram into your precious few hours of 'free' time, when you could be doing something much more fulfilling, perhaps you can work to improve the situation. Try starting to teach the brain injured person where certain items belong, drawing a plan together at home, and getting them to fill in where some of your favourite items are shelved. Then your loved one can have certain things it is their task to go and find. Keep trying, and sense the achievement of planning the shopping task, getting to the supermarket and mixing with other people rather than remaining holed up at home. Give yourself credit for facing up to an ordeal. Another idea is simply to shop online.

It may be that you couldn't enjoy a full-blown meal in a restaurant because the brain injured person would become impatient, or because their behaviour or loud conversation would embarrass you. But you might be able to share a Knickerbocker Glory in an ice-cream parlour and count that as a treat instead.

Perhaps you could manage part of an evening in a pub with friends (before it gets too busy) though you may need to make the compromise of taking a puzzle book along. Perhaps it is unconventional – but does that really matter? You would have gained a social event, and you'd both have had an escape from the house.

In order to claim your own life in and among theirs you will also need to learn how to switch off from embarrassment. Some people hardly know what embarrassment is. Try to take a leaf out of their book. After all, embarrassment in this context is not a helpful emotion; that is, it's not serving to modify anyone's behaviour in line with society's codes. If you let it have the upper hand it will cripple you. You have a range of better ways to deal with a potentially embarrassing situation: you can laugh it off, you can brazen it out, you can explain the reasons for it. And you *can* simply refuse to be embarrassed. Harder than it sounds perhaps, but with practice it does get easier.

You need too to learn how to switch off irritation, by focusing your mind on something else. Embarrassment and irritation are the two emotions that will stand most strongly in the way of your own quality of life. You have much to gain if you can learn to live without them. But beware of slipping into a mode where nothing matters, into the life of the depressive on whom nothing has an impact. Strive to deal with these tensions *for so long*. And then you need to find a way to get away from them.

# *Recognizing your need for support*

If people's difficulties are visible it seems easier for us to cope with them. Epileptic fits draw a sympathetic response. We understand the difficulties of someone with a leg in a plaster cast using crutches to walk. Yes, over time we may get impatient with them, but we can argue back with ourselves. We can also predict what the problems will be in any given situation. The difficulties are measurable, visible, recognized and understood by other people met during the course of the day.

Difficulties that relate to thinking are none of these things. Because thinking is open-ended, endlessly variable according to the endless variety of situations that we find ourselves in, the difficulties are immeasurable. Thinking is invisible. Occasionally, we may get a glimmer of what is going on in someone's mind – see 'light dawn' or read puzzlement in their expression – but we can never be sure, at least not until they choose to express their thoughts and only then if they can do so clearly. Perhaps because we take our thought processes for granted, difficulties with thinking are hard to recognize, especially if there is a conflict between someone looking 'normal' but behaving 'strangely'. Particularly if brain injury is outside the onlooker's experience, it is very hard for them to appreciate what the difficulties might be.

Similarly, it's obvious to everyone that it's hard work looking after someone who is physically disabled. There's no question that, from time to time, the carer will need a break from the physical hard labour. And one of the first to appreciate that need is the one being cared for.

It's much harder to acknowledge the need for respite when there is little or no physical care involved. In this case the stresses and strains are hard to pin down. Hard too when the person being cared for doesn't have proper insight into their own difficulties, let alone the difficulty that they inflict on others.

But stresses and strains there are, however much you might try to dismiss them. In themselves they seem small. The repetitions; you should be used to them by now. The memory difficulties; it's not their fault. The names they call you; they don't mean anything by it.

Even you may scarcely notice the various calls made upon you and the range of tensions you are living with; you have become so used to them. But it is likely that they are causing friction at some level, so that in your day-to-day life when you think you are relaxed, you are probably at a higher level of stress than you realize.

The repetitious questions caused by their memory difficulties try your patience. Their behaviour in public wears you down. Their continuous expressions of undying love make you want to hurl something at them just to stop the record. Their need for a structured routine grates with your need for variety – or just for a lie-in occasionally. And it is quite possible that no one else is thinking to tell you that you need a break, because unless you are living in that situation the stresses and strains of it are not very obvious.

## Developing a support network

In normal circumstances everybody has an off day every once in a while and people have different ways of coping. Some go for a slow, hot bath, treat themselves to a half-hour painting their nails, indulge in a rubbishy magazine or a game of table football, or simply switch off in front of the telly. If none of those work, the next stage might be the whinging phone call to mother or best friend, or going for a drink with a mate.

If it is simply an off day, something as simple as this should do the trick. But sometimes you may feel in need of more support. Different types of support may be wanted at different times. You may want emotional support – someone to pour things out to, perhaps to give you some encouragement and spur you on for the next stage. You may need practical support – someone to have the kids while you take your wife to an appointment, someone to walk the dog for you for a few days so you can catch up on some sleep. Sometimes practical support is needed to bolster your emotional state, and sometimes emotional support is needed to renew your energies to carry out all the practical tasks that are weighing you down.

Different levels of support might be needed at different times. A brief break, or a long holiday. And sometimes you need to be ready to accept support when you don't feel you need it. It may be that the benefit of a break will prevent the tension building up in the first place to the point where you are desperate. Or it may be that if respite provision allocated to you is not used, it will be assumed that you don't need it and it may be passed on to someone else. Then when you do need it and look for it, it may not be available.

You may find after a time that emotional support is difficult for you to access – not because it is not available, but because of your particular circumstances. Normal relationships go through their ups and downs. Someone may pour out their sorrows or complaints to a friend, and after a period of time things will have moved on, the situation will have changed and they will be telling them a further instalment or a different story. Living long-term with a brain injury, though, it is likely that you are going to be wound up by the same things, time after time. Even during the 'early' months, things are moving so very slowly that it is hard to give new news. You might find it hard to be forever complaining about the same things to a friend, or to be always getting upset on them, or burdening them with something they can do nothing about. After a while you are quite likely to feel that you are putting a strain on that friendship.

So you might feel that you want to look beyond your immediate circle of friends and family for some support. If you know other carers in the locality it may be that you can get together socially for informal support, or sometimes share the caring role to give each other a break, depending of course very much on individual circumstances. There may already be such a group in operation, or you might consider starting one.

You may want to join some local or national support group, such as Headway, the Stroke Association or the Encephalitis Society. Sometimes groups offer day centres or similar facilities, social gatherings or educational events. Some groups offer a network, linking sufferers and or carers in similar situations for the purpose of mutual support and ideas and information swapping.

You may be lucky enough to live in an area where Crossroads is active. Crossroads is a charitable organization that has been providing 'in the home care for carers' for 30 years now. If Crossroads doesn't operate locally to you, it may be that the local social services have something of their own to offer, or that there is some other voluntary agency.

The Princess Royal Trust for Carers and Carers UK are two national agencies that exist solely to support carers. The first has a bias towards offering emotional support and, if you have access to the Internet, you can make use of their chatroom and noticeboard where people can link up to support each other and share suggestions based on experience. The second organization is more concerned with campaigning for better recognition and rights. Both offer much useful information.

Since the Carers and Disabled Children's Act was passed in 2000, social services have had a duty to offer a 'carer's assessment', helping the carer consider what support they need and what form that support should take. In a private interview you are able to put forward your views about your situation, particularly about any difficulties that you may be experiencing as a carer. Social services are not allowed to assume that as a carer you are willing to continue caring, or to continue giving the same level of support. But clearly there is an interest in enabling you to continue in that role provided it is to the benefit of all involved. As a result of the assessment, social services will decide what services can be provided, covering such things as emotional support, practical help and short-term breaks from the caring role.

Sometimes, though the support network is there, persuading yourself to make use of it is difficult. You could try asking yourself the following questions:

- Are you trying to prove something to yourself, or to others – and if so, what?
- Are you frightened of the deep-down effect that respite might have on your relationship/on your loved one?
- Do you feel guilty about taking a break, and if so, why?
- What is it that is stopping you from asking for/accepting help?
- Before the injury would you have opportunities to go off and do your own thing and use these, guilt-free? Wouldn't your loved one (*as they really are*) prefer you to do that now?

It can be helpful to remind yourself of the person you are caring for. You know what their difficulties are now, but try to remind yourself of the person they used to be. How would they have coped if they had been left looking after you, instead of vice versa? If that person was also present now, how would they be looking after you? Wouldn't they be encouraging you to take a break, to treat yourself in some way, to look after yourself because you are precious? You owe it to them to take that responsibility for yourself.

# 11

## Listening out

### *Warning signs*

Well, congratulations, you've managed to lift off in your reconstructed life. Here you are, the two of you, still together after the incredible hiatus of a brain injury, coping with all the difficulties it has left in its wake. Normal life has resumed – although not of course the normal life you had before. The brain injury is gradually fading into the past, an accepted fact of your life, and you find that your mind is, on the whole, now preoccupied with other things. A healthy state of affairs.

Or it may be that it's only from the outside that it looks as though everything is fine. Perhaps you put up a good show. After two or more years of being in a state of constant flux, dealing with serious health worries and major domestic upheaval, it may well be that you wearied of 'making a fuss' about your situation. Afraid that the constant 'moaning' might be putting other vital relationships under pressure, perhaps you decided just to shut up.

Nobody looking on can know what a relationship is like on the inside. People – even the brain injured – can be very different in private. Only you can know what the stresses and strains are. Even if many of your loved one's difficulties are obvious, these things impact on different people in different ways. Only you can really know what your life is like and how you are coping with it.

Except that sometimes you don't. We have less insight into our own behaviour than we realize. If you are the sort who just buckles down and gets on with what needs doing, you may not even realize just how much stress you are under, until something finally gives. And then it may be too late, and another crash landing will be inevitable.

Try to develop the habit of living with one ear tuned to the noise of the engine. Without becoming anxious or obsessive about it, just keep an eye on yourself. Are you sleeping okay? Do you feel relaxed when you should? How's your temper? Are you capable of having a good laugh?

If the answers to these things begin to creep towards the negative, perhaps it's a sign that you need a break. Or that you need to have a good moan to someone and get it all off your chest. You need to look after yourself too – for both your sakes.

You may – for the simple reason that it is easier in your circumstances – have got into the habit of shutting yourselves away. Fight against this. We are social animals, designed for living in communities, better able to look out for each other than for ourselves, which is one very good reason for getting involved in a mutual support group. This may be a carers' group set up by the local social services, or a self-help group of brain injured people and their carers, run perhaps under the auspices of Headway. It may even be a church fellowship, a running or art group – nothing whatsoever to do with your caring role.

## Being open to change and taking risks

Not only are we social animals, we are creative animals too. One of the hardest things to cope with in your new life may be the sense that this is it now, your life is fixed. Whereas before the two of you would have had new ideas, new projects and dreams to bring into fruition, this other person in your life now prefers things to stay as they know them, routine and predictable.

Although this may go against the grain, at the same time, because it demands less of you, it is easy to fall in with. Try not to. You must have dreams to keep you going. You must have variety and change to keep you properly alive.

The routine and structure that your loved one needs is actually more of a backcloth than the stage itself. You are yourself probably the mainstay of that structure and so long as you are there, she will cope with other changes. In fact, change may have much less impact than we anticipate. Because change – moving house, for example – is stressful for ourselves, we expect it to be extremely difficult for the brain injured. But if awareness of the environment is reduced, she may sail through with the change going almost unnoticed.

We need to take risks too. Without taking risks in life we never grow, never learn. Not only do you need to keep growing, keep learning, so does your loved one, albeit at a much slower rate. Yes, there will be opportunities that you turn down as too difficult to handle with a brain injury to consider. But try not to do this too often. Simply because something has been problematic before does not mean it will necessarily be so for ever. If you close your mind to it, all that can result is a sense of disgruntlement and frustration. The passage of time, a little bit more healing, more adjustment, may have made a difference without you becoming aware of it. Take this risk, give it a try and you may find you have managed to win yourself some positive encouragement. At the very least, you can congratulate yourself on being prepared to live dangerously.

## Keeping in touch with new developments and research

The brain is currently one of the main frontiers of scientific and medical research. Perhaps because of the large numbers of people now living with a brain injury, there is much popular interest in this field too. You may feel that understanding of how the brain works is actually of little interest; what is needed is understanding of how to mend malfunctioning parts, or replace parts that have died. Perhaps the time will come when that too will be possible. Meanwhile, this is a step on the way and without keeping an open mind and an ear to the ground you will never know if you have missed something that might have been useful to you.

Membership of one of the brain injury associations (see 'Useful addresses') will help in this way. The pooling of information is the only way in which the human race can make progress. All the associations are involved in research of some kind to some extent, and from time to time they ask for volunteers who are willing to help with research projects, whether by answering questionnaires or undergoing tests of some sort. Each association also acts as a forum for ideas and experiences where people can share success stories, express their frustration or ask for help in overcoming particular difficulties.

You didn't wish for this event in your life, but it happened. However much you regret your experiences, they may be of help to someone else. Perhaps now that you have regained some stability you might be able to offer a helping hand to someone further back on the road, whether by a one-to-one contact through a support group, by answering a plea for help in a newsletter or by offering your experiences for a research programme. You too have your contribution to make.

# Useful addresses

## *Brain injury associations*

**Acquire**
Manor Farm House, Wendlebury, Bicester OX25 2PW
Tel: 01869 324339
Website: www.acquire.org.uk
Email: info@acquire.org.uk
(Focuses on the educational needs of adults, young people and children with acquired brain injury.)

**Brain and Spine Injury Charity (BASIC)**
The Neurocare Centre, 554 Eccles New Road, Salford M5 1AL
Tel: 0161 707 6441
Website: www.basiccharity.org.uk
Email: enquiries@basiccharity.org.uk
(Raising funds for research into the brain since 1986, BASIC has more recently extended its services to include support and information for those recovering from a life-threatening condition affecting the brain or spine.)

**Brain Injury Rehabilitation Trust**
Hallcroft House, 24 Castleford Road, Normanton, Wakefield WF6 2DW
Tel: 01924 896100
Website: www.birt.co.uk
Email: birt@disabilities-trust.org.uk
(Europe's largest independent provider of brain injury rehabilitation services.)

**British Brain and Spine Foundation**
7 Winchester House, Kennington Park, Cranmer Road
London SW9 6EJ
Tel: 020 7793 5900
Website: www.bbsf.org.uk

(Set up in 1992 to develop research, education and information programmes aimed at improving the prevention, treatment and care of people affected by disorders of the brain and spine.)

**Encephalitis Society**
7b Saville Street, Malton, North Yorkshire YO17 7LL
Tel: 01653 692583 (Admin); 01653 699599 (Support)
Website: www.encephalitis.info
Email: mail@encephalitis.info
(Working to improve the quality of life of all people directly and indirectly affected by encephalitis.)

**Headway**
Tel: 0115 924 0800
Freephone Helpline: 0808 800 2244 (9 a.m. – 5 p.m., Monday to Friday)
Website: www.headway.org.uk
Email: enquiries@headway.org.uk
(A national association with over 100 local Headway groups and branches across the UK, offering support for people with brain injury, their families, carers and those working with them.)

**Rehab UK**
Windermere House, Kendal Avenue, London W3 0XA
Tel: 020 8896 2333
Website: www.rehabuk.org
Email: info@rehabuk.org
(Provides assessment, training and development programmes that enable people with disabilities to break into the workforce. Operates a network of brain injury centres.)

**Stroke Association**
Stroke House, 240 City Road, London EC1V 2PR
Tel: 020 7566 0300
Helpline: 0845 303 3100
Website: www.stroke.org.uk
Email: info@stroke.org.uk
(Has 16 regional centres and over 400 affiliated stroke clubs throughout the country.)

# Carers' associations

**Carers UK**
20/25 Glasshouse Yard, London EC1A 4JT
Tel: 020 7490 8818
Website: www.carersonline.org.uk
Email: info@carersuk.org

**Crossroads Association**
10 Regent Place, Rugby, Warwickshire CV21 2PN
Tel: 0845 450 0350
Website: www.crossroads.org.uk
Email: communications@crossroads.org.uk

**Princess Royal Trust for Carers**
142 Minories, London EC3N 1LB
Tel: 020 7480 7788
Website: www.carers.org
Email: info@carers.org or help@carers.org

## Governmental information

For information on the Government's National Strategy for Carers:
www.carers.gov.uk
For comprehensive information on benefits: www.dwp.gov.uk

# Driving

**Driver and Vehicle Licensing Authority (DVLA)**
Longview Road, Swansea SA6 7JL
Tel: 01792 782341
Website: www.dvla.gov.uk

**Motability Operations**
City Gate House, 22 Southwark Bridge Road, London SE1 9HB
Tel: 0845 456 4566
Website: www.motability.co.uk
(An independent not-for-profit organization which provides mobility
solutions for disabled people, including those who cannot drive
themselves.)

# Index